HARDWIRED
FOR FITNESS

The evolutionary way to lose weight, have more
energy, and improve body composition—naturally.

Robert Portman, Ph.D.
and John Ivy, Ph.D.

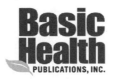

Basic Health
Health
PUBLICATIONS, INC.

The information contained in this book is based upon the research and personal and professional experiences of the authors. It is not intended as a substitute for consulting with your physician or other healthcare provider. Any attempt to diagnose and treat an illness should be done under the direction of a healthcare professional.

The publisher does not advocate the use of any particular healthcare protocol but believes the information in this book should be available to the public. The publisher and authors are not responsible for any adverse effects or consequences resulting from the use of the suggestions, preparations, or procedures discussed in this book. Should the reader have any questions concerning the appropriateness of any procedures or preparation mentioned, the authors and the publisher strongly suggest consulting a professional healthcare advisor.

Basic Health Publications, Inc.
28812 Top of the World Drive
Laguna Beach, CA 92651
949-715-7327 • www.basichealthpub.com

Library of Congress Cataloging-in-Publication Data

Library of Congress Cataloging-in-Publication Data is available through the Library of Congress.

Editor: Cheryl Hirsch
Typesetting/Book design: Gary A. Rosenberg
Cover design: Andrea Jennings

Printed in the United States of America

10   9   8   7   6   5   4   3   2   1

Contents

Acknowledgments

We would first like to acknowledge the many scientists whose brilliant studies and insights provided the underpinnings for this book. We are also grateful to the many people who provided valuable suggestions and comments. Special thanks to Nancy Marshello, who managed to keep the project on track in spite of multiple distractions. Special acknowledgement should also go to Brittany Crim, our knowledgeable registered dietitian, who created easy-to-follow healthy and delicious recipes based on unique calorie and macronutrient requirements.

We would like to acknowledge Norman Goldfind, publisher of Basic Health Publications, who has consistently been an enthusiastic supporter of each and every new book project. Special gratitude to Cheryl Hirsch, whose patience, insights, and criticisms created a far more readable book. We would like to also acknowledge Jon Portman for creating the special art that appears throughout the book and Andrea Jennings for her brilliant cover design.

Finally, we would like to thank our wives, Jennifer and Susan, whose enthusiasm for the project has never waned.

Preface

We have conducted research in the area of fitness and weight management for more than 50 years combined. Therefore, it's surprising that the origins of this book did not evolve from studies with overweight and out-of-shape people. Rather, the origins emanated from research we, along with other colleagues, have conducted with elite athletes. These athletes had the body compositions most of us only dream about: 6 to 8 percent body fat for men and 12 to 16 percent for women. The average American has a considerably higher body fat composition. These athletes also had extraordinary endurance capacity and strength.

Our research focused on improving the athlete's capacity to recover after a strenuous high-intensity workout. Following a hard workout, muscle energy stores are depleted and muscle protein is damaged. An athlete's ability to perform at an optimum level in the next workout depends on how quickly his or her muscles recover. We designed our studies to determine if different nutrient-rich beverages could improve the quality and speed of the recovery process. To our initial surprise, we observed that *when* a beverage was consumed played a critical role in whether it had an effect. If the beverage was consumed immediately after exercise, there were significant benefits in terms of replenishing energy stores, and repairing and rebuilding muscle protein.

When a recovery beverage was consumed two hours after exercise, it had almost no effect. It was as if a switch that activated the muscle's metabolic machinery was turned on after exercise, and two hours later the switch was turned off. Further studies revealed that this was exactly what was happening. After exercise, the pathways that rebuild the muscles and their vital energy stores were activated. Providing a nutritionally rich beverage at this time produced extraordinary benefits. We refer to this interval after exercise as the "metabolic window of opportunity."

The Metabolic Window of Opportunity

The athletes who participated in these studies were already adhering to a training regimen that optimized performance. They consumed a healthy diet that contained sufficient protein plus an abundance of fruits and vegetables, and followed the latest training techniques. We expected that any benefits resulting from taking advantage of the metabolic window through postexercise nutrition would be small, but they were not: the benefits were *huge*.

We discovered that postexercise nutrition reduced residual muscle damage by up to 90 percent and improved endurance performance as much as 36 percent in a second exercise bout conducted *18 hours later*. Other research studies also confirmed that postexercise nutrition consumed when the metabolic window was open stimulated the breakdown of fat and increased the manufacture of lean body mass. Obviously, powerful mechanisms were at work. It was also logical to conclude that only super-fit individuals had the capacity for this unique metabolic adaptation.

However, in 2001, a group of Danish researchers published a fascinating study in which the participants were as far from elite athletes as possible. The study investigated the timing of after-exercise beverages on muscle recovery in 74-year-old men. The exercise consisted of a modest 12-week program of resistance training three times a week. One group consumed the beverage immediately after exercise, while the second group drank the beverage two hours later.

Taken in context, the results achieved with these senior "athletes" were equally as impressive as those seen with our elite endurance athletes. The Danish researchers reported a significant increase in muscle growth and strength in the group who consumed the recovery drink immediately after exercise compared with the group who drank it two hours after exercise. We could only conclude that the metabolic window of opportunity was clearly not a phenomenon limited to athletes; rather, the programming that controlled this interval was hardwired into our DNA.

Metabolic Pathways Became Ultra-Efficient

It was apparent from the studies with the elite athletes and seniors that in order for the metabolic benefits to occur, three essential conditions had to be present: physical activity, timing of nutrition, and a specific combination of nutrients. In the presence of all three, the metabolic machinery went into an ultra-efficient mode that impacted both the speed and the quality of the muscle recovery process.

These findings ultimately became the basis of our book *Nutrient Timing* (Basic Health Publications, 2004). Since that time, hundreds of research papers have confirmed that the timing of nutrient consumption is a critical component in improving athletic performance. Postexercise recovery nutrition has become an essential part of the training regimen for athletes at all levels, from high school to college, from professionals to Olympians, as well as for ordinary people who regularly exercise.

We Are Not Born to Exercise

The results of our research on nutrient timing raised intriguing philosophical, scientific, and practical questions. The fact that our DNA contains the programming that switches on this metabolic machinery after exercise is somewhat puzzling. Adaptations that are incorporated into human DNA occur over hundreds of thousands, and possibly millions, of years.

Archaeologists who sift through the soil in an attempt to define the life - styles of our Paleolithic ancestors do not find treadmills or exercise bikes among the primitive hunting tools and cooking implements, and for good reason. Exercise is a relatively recent activity in human history and is not a natural part of our makeup. Paleolithic man did not exercise. He was a hunter-gatherer who was on the move most of the day, but his activities were not pre-designed to develop fitness. While the Greeks certainly admired exercise and fitness, and built games around them, it was more for the sake of competition and entertainment rather than for "staying in shape."

Exercise, as we know it today, is still not a part of the lifestyle of the majority of people in the world. In fact, 90 percent of the world's population does not participate in formal exercise. In the United States, according to the Centers for Disease Control and Prevention (CDC), only 25 percent of the population exercises regularly. What most of the world's population has in common with our Paleolithic ancestors is that their lifestyle and working routine forces them to be physically active throughout the day.

So, why are there specific adaptations within our genes that are keyed to exercise recovery? The answer is that these adaptations had nothing to do with exercise. There was an evolutionary advantage for Paleolithic man to recover quickly after an intense burst of aerobic activity, such as hunting for dinner. Failure to recover quickly would have made him more vulnerable to dangerous prey. The existence of a metabolic window following exercise raised the intriguing possibility that, during our daily 24-hour cycle, there are other metabolic windows, or specific functional intervals, where our metabolic machinery could be activated, causing a major impact on how our bodies perform and adapt to a variety of environmental influences.

If these intervals could be turned on as easily as a postexercise switch, and they delivered similar physiological and metabolic benefits, we would have discovered the "Holy Grail" for fitness. First, however, we would have to (1) identify the functional intervals, (2) identify the switches that control them, and (3) once the switches are turned on, determine how to optimize their effects.

For example, we found that although a carbohydrate or a protein recovery drink improved recovery when consumed immediately after exercise, neither was anywhere near as effective as a drink that contained a mixture of carbohydrate and protein. This was critically important, because even though our DNA controlled the timing of the functional interval, the nutritional composition of the beverage is what determined the magnitude of the response. To get full benefit of the functional interval, the right combination of nutrients had to be consumed at the right time.

We discovered that one of the most important aspects of the postexercise functional interval was that it does not require an extraordinary effort on the part of the athlete in order to receive its full benefit. Most athletes normally eat within two to three hours after a workout. In the past, their postexercise meal might have consisted of a protein drink or a meal of mixed macronutrients. But once we defined the nature of the functional interval, the recommendations we made for the athletes were quite simple: eat foods or beverages that contain the right macronutrient composition within 30 to 45 minutes after exercising, and you will maximize your rate of recovery. There was almost no disruption of the athletes' training regimens or normal eating patterns.

Throughout our years of research into nutrition and fitness, we have learned that unless compliance to a fitness program is easy, it will generally fail. This means that a program must be compatible with a person's lifestyle. Most diets or exercise programs are not successful long-term because one's lifestyle isn't taken into account or the regimen called for is too strenuous (more on this later). The fact that the benefits of the postexercise functional interval can be achieved with almost no change in a person's lifestyle makes it a potent tool. Commitment follows naturally if changes in daily routines bring about a desired effect naturally and conveniently.

Are We Born to Be Fit?

Although we were aware that exercise opened the metabolic recovery interval, we knew that it had to work through a specific metabolic switch or a metabolic switching system. The enormous benefits derived from consuming a recovery drink postexercise did not come from activation of a single metabolic pathway. We knew, for example, that restoration of muscle energy stores and repair of damaged muscle protein were controlled by discrete metabolic pathways. Therefore, the switch had to have the capacity to turn on multiple pathways that restored, repaired, and rebuilt the muscle cell while simultaneously turning off the pathways that may have caused further fuel depletion and damage. Once the switch was identified, we could then explain why certain combinations of macronutrients were better than others. The implication that multiple functional intervals are programmed into our DNA is immense, especially as it relates to fitness.

For the past 50 years, exercise physiologists have defined fitness in terms of body weight, body composition, and activity capacity (the ability to perform daily activities without fatigue and to respond to situations that require high-energy expenditure). In this book, we define the physiological circuits that determine whether we are fit or out of shape. Our level of fitness is the composite activity of four essential circuits: energy, appetite, stress, and protein turnover. What exercise physiologists didn't have was a full understanding of the switches that turn these key circuits on and off, how these circuits are programmed, and the influence of diet, physical activity, sleep, and timing of meals.

We began an odyssey that involved our own original research, as well as a search of the scientific literature. We found long-forgotten studies that helped explain why fitness has become such a difficult goal to achieve for most Americans, and we were aided by cutting-edge research that helped define the key switches that control fitness. What we discovered is that *our bodies are hardwired to be fit*. In the process, we recognized why so much of the prevailing dogma regarding weight loss and fitness is simply wrong. Our bodies have functional intervals hardwired into our DNA. This hardwiring controls our weight, our body composition, and our capacity to be active—in other words, our fitness level. Our bodies are programmed to maintain a critical level of fitness. Nutrition, meal timing, and specific environmental factors influence when and whether these master switches are turned on and off. The unmistakable conclusion is that we are born to be fit.

Hardwired for Fitness explains what the key fitness circuits are, how they can be rewired so that they work as intended, and what foods and activities can best switch them on and off. So, if you are a person who has tried and failed on many occasions to lose weight and get into shape, or has refused to even start a program because it seems too daunting, or is in shape but wants to get to the next level, this book will show you how to achieve your goal in a natural and stress-free way.

Introduction

We are hardwired to be fit and lean. This will come as a shock to the tens of millions of people who struggle to get in shape and, as a result of their struggles, have created a multibillion-dollar fitness and weight-loss industry encompassing food, diet plans, exercise equipment, and celebrity-authored diet books and supplements. Despite this obsession, Americans are not only losing the battle but we're becoming more desperate as well.

"The Diet Product Is a Success, But You're a Failure"

Meeting consumer expectation is a fundamental marketing principle in determining whether a product is a commercial success. Any overweight person who has purchased a diet book or enrolled in a diet plan has the expectation of long-term weight loss. "This time I'll lose the weight and keep it off," or so they think. The diet industry is unique in the consumer world, especially in the Internet age, where dissatisfied consumers have an instant forum to publicize their product experiences. At best, these products deliver short- or intermediate-term weight loss of 10 to 20 percent. They almost never produce permanent weight loss. And when the product does fail, disappointed consumers generally don't fault the product but rather blame themselves: "I didn't have the willpower," "I was traveling," "I was depressed," "I'm going through a difficult time at work." The consumer then buys another diet product or plan, and the cycle continues—much to the joy of the diet industry.

It is estimated that at any given time almost 120 million Americans are dieting. Liposuction has now become one of the most commonly performed surgical procedures. And here is the most depressing fact of all: People who diet regularly are more likely to experience weight gain.

In 2007, researchers at the University of California, Los Angeles (UCLA), published a study that confirmed what almost every person who has ever gone on a diet has discovered through personal experience. The researchers analyzed 31 long-term weight-loss studies involving 19,000 subjects and found that people on diets typically lose 5 to 10 percent of their beginning weight in the first six months. The overwhelming majority actually regained *more* weight than they lost within three to five years. The authors made three important conclusions: (1) dieting doesn't work, (2) people who don't diet gain less weight over the long-term than people who do, and (3) previous dieting is an accurate predictor of future weight gain.

In other words, this study suggests that dieting may be a primary cause for the increased incidence of obesity in our country. After the results were published, a prominent physician who specialized in weight loss was quoted as saying: "There might be benefits in losing weight for a period of time even if you regain it than not having lost the weight at all." Based on the number of studies documenting the increased risks of serial dieting, we wonder on which planet this physician is practicing.

"It's in My Genes"

In 1994, researchers at Rockefeller University discovered leptin, a protein found in adipose (fat) tissue of mice that were genetically bred for obesity. These mice had voracious appetites and very low leptin levels. Subsequent studies showed that leptin is an important signal in controlling body weight through appetite and energy expenditure. This discovery generated a great deal of excitement. The media suggested that researchers had finally found the cure for obesity. However, the promise of leptin as a weight-loss tool did not pan out. Studies with obese people showed that they had higher than normal levels of leptin and administration of leptin had little impact on appetite or energy expenditure. But the discovery of leptin did represent a defining moment in our understanding of obesity because it shed light on genetic mechanisms that impact appetite and energy expenditure. It also stimulated extensive research by pharmaceutical companies to identify other molecules that influence weight and energy expenditure. This has been a tried-and-true approach to the development of innovative drugs. Understanding the genetic mechanisms of many diseases has resulted in novel and effective therapies.

Although this approach may result in drugs that produce short-term weight loss, it is highly unlikely that drugs will ever become the magic bullet people are seeking. Food consumption and energy expenditure are part of an integrated group of pathways or circuits. The functioning of these circuits is fundamental to our survival and a million years of evolution have made them extremely efficient. When a person interferes with a specific circuit such as appetite, as you will learn, it causes a counter response by the body that ultimately leads to weight-loss failure.

A second part of the genetic argument is that people are overweight because of their genes. Genetics has become an appealing reason to explain the increase in obesity and lack of fitness. The argument goes as follows: The genetic composition of certain people is such that when placed in a potentially negative food environment, they respond differently. In other words, two people exposed to plentiful amounts of fast food will respond differently because of their genetic composition. If you are unfortunate enough to have a fat gene, you will gain far more weight than somebody who doesn't. It's unfortunate that this argument is given credence by well-known molecular biologists. It simply ignores genetics. It is implausible to suggest that, as human beings evolved, genetic adaptations were created in our DNA anticipating that 1 million years later fast-food establishments would litter the landscape. Quite the contrary, principles of genetics suggest that when adaptations are not used, they are lost.

Adding to the implausibility of the "it's in my genes" rationale is that the largest increase in obesity has occurred within the last 25 years, a time when most of the people who are obese today were alive. Although we do not have accurate data of body fat percentages extending back thousands of years, the data that we do have indicate that the percentage of obese people in the population did not change between 1800 and 1950 and was estimated to be 3 percent. Even the most radical geneticists would agree that

50 years is insufficient to produce a genetic adaptation. There is little doubt that our genetic disposition influences our fitness level, but it is an intellectual stretch to say that the increased percentage of obesity is primarily the result of genetic factors.

The Sisyphean Frustration

In Greek mythology a king named Sisyphus, from the ancient kingdom of Corinth, angered Zeus and was sentenced to a lifetime of pushing a large boulder up a mountain. Each time the boulder neared the top, it would roll back down, and Sisyphus had to start pushing anew. In many ways, the travails of Sisyphus describe the estimated 120 million Americans who are dieting at any given moment. It takes a great deal of willpower and energy to lose weight, which is analogous to pushing a large boulder up a mountain (Figure 1). Statistics show that very few people are successful in reaching the summit. A more common scenario is that they almost get to the summit, stop and take a break, and the boulder rolls downhill—where it remains until they start their next fitness or weight-loss program. The reason it is so difficult to reach the fitness summit is that conventional, popular, and unconventional fitness and weight-loss programs work against

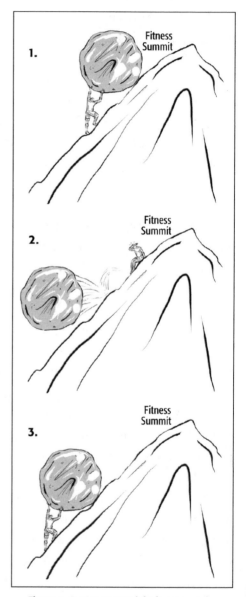

Figure 1. A common weight-loss scenario.

the body's natural physiological rhythm. The few people who manage to reach the summit are a testament to the power of will and personal commitment.

New Miracle Fitness Product

The desperation to be thin is exploited by the thousands of companies that sell products ranging from weight-loss creams and supplements to meal plans and abdominal crunchers. All the products have a common denominator: they are touted as the next "miracle" that will transform an out-of-shape, overweight person into the perfection of fitness. The sheer number and variety of programs and products that populate this category suggest that one should be the next miracle. After wasting time, money, and hope, consumers find there is no such thing as a miracle. Depending on the company's budget, each has its 15 minutes of fame, and the disenchanted public looks for the next miracle.

Now let's suppose you are one of the millions of overweight and out-of-shape people who have read about a new fitness product that claimed the following:

- Guaranteed to help you lose weight, improve body composition, and give you more energy
- Safety proven in more than 1 million years of continuous use
- All natural
- No side effects
- Used successfully by billions of people
- Proven effective in thousands of studies
- Is absolutely free

You would probably be lining up to receive this product, while the Federal Trade Commission (FTC), which monitors advertising of weight-loss and fitness products, would be preparing to have the product removed from the market for making outrageous claims. Such a product does exist, and it provides even greater benefits than the ones highlighted above. And, the FTC cannot remove it from the market.

The product that we describe above exists within our own DNA. Our DNA contains specific genes that program essential circuits or pathways that determine our level of fitness. In this book, you'll learn how this programming works and how, over the short span of 50 years, through changes in eating, lifestyle, and activity patterns, we have managed to disconnect key circuits, causing a high percentage of the population to become overweight and out of shape.

Fitness Wasn't an Alternative

For more than 1 million years, the programming in our DNA maintained our weight at an optimal level, created the lean body mass necessary for us to perform essential physical tasks, and provided the adaptations necessary to maintain a very physical existence—in other words, to keep us fit. For our Paleolithic ancestors, fitness was not defined in terms of how they looked, how they competed in athletic competition, or what size clothing they wore. Fitness was a matter of survival. Nature could not depend solely on the savvy or resourcefulness of early man to survive. Without being fit, the human race would have become extinct eons ago. The metabolic adaptations that permitted our Paleolithic ancestors not only to survive, but also to flourish, were programmed into their DNA—a very similar DNA to that found in our cells today.

This should not be surprising. It is the core principle of evolution. Charles Darwin said that in true natural selection or survival of the fittest, it is the genes or DNA that give organisms the qualities that enable them to survive. In the search for fitness and weight-loss miracles, we have ignored this fundamental observation.

There is much pessimism about why it is so difficult for people to lose weight and get in shape. Experts say the problem resides within us—our metabolism is slow or our hormones are out of balance, or perhaps our diet is wrong or we lack willpower. All these reasons lose sight of the fact that the body's fitness circuitry is a remarkable, integrated piece of engineering. It has worked incredibly well for more than 1 million years, and it can work for another million years if we simply implement a few simple measures to resynchronize and reconnect the circuitry.

The body's fitness circuitry is amazing in another way. It does not require much attention on our part to work optimally. It is almost maintenance free, and anytime our actions place undue hardship on one or more of the circuits, they have the ability to compensate for a short time and keep the body functioning normally. However, this compensation cannot continue indefinitely without unwanted consequences. Fortunately, these fitness circuits can be resynchronized with little effort and our fitness restored naturally. Paleolithic man did not have the time to worry about fitness. It just happened because of his natural lifestyle. This book will show you how to just make it happen too. You will learn about the master switches that control your fitness circuits, and how, through minimal lifestyle changes, you can reprogram these switches and reconnect your circuits to give you the level of fitness you have always wanted.

Fit or Fat?

In the 1970s, a popular book was published that suggested that you could either be fit *or* fat. Through the years, this proposition has been adopted by health professionals and has become a popular talking point by politicians. "Overweight" and "obesity" are synonymous for being out of shape and unfit. Today, as the debate for an overhaul of our health system takes center stage, the problem of obesity in this country has reached near hysterical levels. Obesity-related disease is said to represent almost 16 percent of overall U.S. healthcare costs.

Multiple studies have shown that obesity increases the risk for many chronic diseases, including diabetes and heart disease, and negatively impacts healthcare costs to the tune of $147 billion per year. However, this focus on obesity loses sight of the more important issue—and that is fitness. Today, a lack of fitness and being overweight/obese are used interchangeably. You are probably asking, "But aren't they the same thing?" They are not. The determination of whether someone is overweight or obese depends on his or her body mass index (BMI).

BMI is an indirect measure of body fat using height and weight. For the vast majority of people, BMI is an accurate reflection of whether they are underweight, normal, overweight, or obese. Although weight is an important component in determining our level of fitness, it is only one component. Using BMI as the sole criteria to define fitness, however, paints a distorted picture of whether an individual is fit or not. It is only one component of the fitness triad.

The two other essential components that compose the fitness triad are percentage of body fat (or body composition) and activity capacity. Percentage of body fat is an indicator of lean body or muscle mass. Body fat is an important predictor of coronary heart disease, other cardiovascular problems, and diseases associated with abnormal metabolic function such as type 2 diabetes. The third component, activity capacity, is a person's ability to perform daily activities without fatigue and to have sufficient capacity to meet short-term energy needs, such as sprinting for the bus, dodging an errant ball, or running away from a dangerous situation.

Our level of fitness, of which BMI is certainly an important component, is a far more accurate determinant of our overall health, and it is also a barometer for future disease risk. The singular focus on BMI or body weight rather than on fitness is one of the major shortcomings of the current health dialogue. The primary message of the healthcare community is that simply losing weight so that your BMI is in the normal range will improve your life and reduce the risk of future disease. That is not only a distortion of the facts, but, as you will learn, a singular focus on weight loss forces you into constant conflict with your body's natural biological rhythm. For the tens of millions of people who have lost weight time and time again only to regain it, this book will show you why success is so rare and how to break this frustrating cycle once and for all.

The parameters that define fitness were established by exercise scientists decades ago. Only recently have the underlying biochemical mechanisms of the body's fitness circuitry been described. Scientists have identified the key master switches and the principal factors that control how they work. This has led to significant breakthroughs in understanding how fitness is programmed into the DNA. The master switches are primarily proteins that have the capacity to determine whether you are hungry or full, whether food should be stored or used as energy, whether protein should be synthesized or broken down, or whether stress levels should be high or low. In other words, your fitness circuitry determines whether you are normal weight, have low body fat, and have the ability to respond to an increased energy need. Scientists have also learned that the switching mechanism has a natural metabolic rhythm throughout the day. Understanding how this metabolic rhythm varies over the course of the day gives you an effective tool for becoming fit.

Our Genetic Clock

The earliest known observation that the body's cycles of sleep and wakefulness match the rotation of the earth was made almost 2,500 years ago when a ship captain named Androsthenes, serving under Alexander the Great, described diurnal (occurring in the daytime) leaf movements of the tamarind tree. Androsthenes noted that the leaves moved in a predictable pattern over 24 hours even when they were placed in a completely dark environment. In other words, the leaf movements were not caused by the changing cycle of light and dark, but rather were internally generated by a mechanism within the DNA of the tamarind leaf. The term used to describe this phenomenon is circadian (about the day) rhythm.

In 1994, scientists discovered that the circadian rhythm in mammals has a genetic basis. Circadian rhythm is the master "clock" that is programmed into the DNA of all living creatures. The circadian clock in mammals is located in a pair of distinct groups of cells located in the hypothalamus, a region of the brain. Anyone who has traveled through multiple time zones in a 24-hour period has certainly felt the effects of a disrupted circadian rhythm—sleeplessness, disorientation, and loss of appetite. What most people don't realize, however, is that circadian rhythm controls more than just sleep and hunger patterns. It coordinates the release of hormones and other metabolic activators, controls metabolic pathways, and regulates eating patterns and physical activity.

Circadian rhythm also synchronizes the many physiological processes that control energy utilization, cellular repair, and appetite. It is the principle control mechanism that has allowed our species to survive and thrive. Just how powerful a force is the circadian rhythm is shown by animal experiments in which artificially interfering with the normal light-dark cycle decreases their longevity.

Our master clock is programmed so that we are physically active during daylight hours and sleep at night. This adaptation was crucial because our senses of smell, hearing, and sight never developed to the level necessary for us to successfully hunt and be active at night. Although our modern lifestyle challenges these nocturnal limitations, our master clock represents a potent force in determining our daily natural metabolic rhythm. As you will learn, the fundamental reason almost every diet or exercise plan fails over the long-term is because it does not take into account the programming of this master clock.

An All-or-Nothing Proposition

We now know that the body's fitness circuits are switched on and off during the course of the day. When these circuits are functioning in harmony, they can activate your metabolic machinery far more effectively and safely than any commercial product. For example, our bodies have the ability to:

• Burn fat more quickly than most expensive thermogenic supplements

• Decrease food intake more effectively than most costly appetite suppressants

• Synthesize protein faster than the leading protein powder

You are probably wondering, "What's the catch?" First, you have to disregard many of the ideas you hold dear about weight loss and fitness, and why you can't get in shape. Second, and most important, you have to understand that the Hardwired Fitness Program is an all-or-nothing proposition. In other words, if you are simply looking to lose weight, this book won't help you, because your body does not contain an independent circuit responsible for weight loss. Neither will this book help you if you are looking only to decrease body fat, because the circuitry responsible for lean body mass is wired into the circuitry that also controls appetite and energy.

Although the Hardwired Fitness Program won't selectively change your body composition or decrease your weight, it will positively impact all three factors that determine your fitness level: BMI, percentage of body fat, and capacity to be active. We can't give you one, but this program can give you all three. Once you are physically fit, you will have the energy necessary to pursue your leisure-time interests and make your day more productive. Being physically fit will strengthen your immune system and reduce your susceptibility to colds and other infectious diseases. Being fit will decrease your risk of developing chronic diseases and it will help you live longer. Fitness is about a better quality of life.

Instead of fighting your body's natural metabolic rhythm or pushing a large boulder uphill, this book will show you how to enlist the powerful traits that exist within your DNA to achieve your fitness goal. In other words, you will be pushing the boulder downhill, because you are working with—rather than against—your body's natural physiological rhythm (Figure 2). You will see results within weeks, and your level of fitness will keep improving over time.

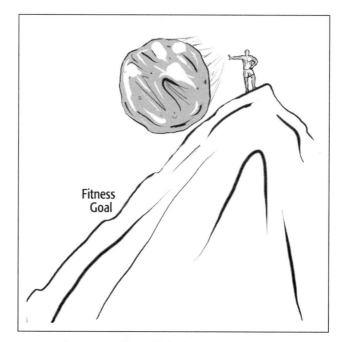

Figure 2. Working with the body's natural rhythm.

PART ONE

Born to Be Fit

If you have embarked on a weight-loss and fitness program and have been unsuccessful, your natural inclination is to say, "My body has failed me." In reality, nothing can be further from the truth. Our ability to survive over millions of years is an undeniable testament to the efficiency and adaptability of the body's metabolic machinery. What has changed, however, particularly over the last 50 years, is the external environment in which this metabolic engine operates. As a result, we have decreased the efficiency of the engine and impaired its natural ability to respond to a wide range of conditions.

Our state of fitness is determined by a highly integrated group of circuits. Altering any one can produce unintended consequences. In Part One, you will learn about these circuits, how they are integrated, what turns them on and off, and why this integration is so essential to achieving and maintaining a level of fitness. You will also learn why much of the conventional wisdom and advice, which ignores the body's natural metabolic rhythm, makes it impossible to achieve long-term fitness. You will discover why extreme dietary regimens and pills can't possibly work, and over the long-term may actually increase weight while decreasing fitness. You will see how we have disconnected this fitness circuitry and why much of the current thinking about weight loss and fitness is simply wrong.

Most important, you will also learn that resynchronizing and restoring the natural balance of the circuits that determine whether you are fit or unfit is neither complicated nor difficult to do.

CHAPTER 1

Survival of the Fittest, Not the Thinnest

(with Apologies to C. Darwin)

A cynical friend asked us why we didn't call this book *Hardwired for Weight Loss*. His reasoning is that most Americans are more concerned with weight loss than fitness. It is hard to argue with this conclusion. We spend more than $100 billion a year looking for a weight-loss miracle that always seems to be just out of reach. Much of our national dialogue focuses on weight loss. The relationships between obesity and risk factors for diabetes and cardiovascular disease are certainly well defined and well publicized.

Despite this intense focus on weight loss, obesity has continued to rise at alarming rates. The latest government statistics show that 66 percent of American adults are either overweight or obese. If we were to analyze the array of products, supplements, diet plans, and programs that are available today, one of them should work simply by the laws of statistical probability. The fact of the matter is that none of them do, because their end point is weight loss not fitness, and a singular focus on weight loss is an impediment to fitness.

IT'S ABOUT METABOLIC EFFICIENCY, NOT CALORIES

Energy efficiency is a dominating topic of interest in our green-conscious society. A major thrust of the green movement is to develop more energy-efficient technology that will give us the same benefit as existing technology but use less energy. Energy efficiency should play an equally prominent

15

role in terms of weight loss and fitness, but, ironically, it is ignored. Anyone who has ever started a diet plan or fitness program is familiar with the
first law of thermodynamics, even if he or she is not familiar with the term.
Simply stated, the first law of thermodynamics describes the conversion of
energy. This law is translated by weight-loss experts into the simple state-
ment: "A calorie is a calorie is a calorie." A calorie of food is equal to a calorie of activity is equal to a calorie of fat.

One pound of body fat contains 3,500 calories; therefore, to lose a
pound, we have to either eat less or move more so we produce a negative
calorie deficit equal to 3,500 calories. As shown in the inset below, when
energy expenditure is equal to energy consumption, we maintain our
weight. When energy consumption is more than energy expenditure we
gain weight. However, when energy consumption is less than energy
expenditure, we lose weight—hence, the can't-miss formula: "Eat less,
move more." By doing both, we are working both ends of the energy equation in our favor.

Eat Less, Move More

Weight Maintenance:	Energy Expenditure = Energy Consumed
Weight Gain:	Energy Expenditure < Energy Consumption
	Energy Consumption > Energy Expenditure
Weight Loss:	Energy Consumption < Energy Expenditure
	Energy Expenditure > Energy Consumption

Although this advice is quite simple, it has made millions of people
who have attempted to follow the principle in real life feel inadequate. It's
exceedingly difficult to do. The problem is that we should be focusing on
the second law of thermodynamics, which is far more representative of
how the body and other sophisticated engines work. The second law con-
cerns the relative efficiency of an engine. For example, if you own a car
and simply follow the first law of thermodynamics, you can reduce the
energy expenditure by putting less fuel in the tank. Unfortunately, this

may not get you to work. A far better approach is to increase the efficiency of the engine so that the same gallon of gas enables you to go 30 miles rather than 15.

This analogy is particularly apt when it comes to weight loss. Almost all diets emphasize reducing consumption rather than creating conditions that increase the efficiency of the body's fitness pathways. This is a far easier task than you might imagine. In the preface, we described research involving two very different populations of subjects, seniors and elite athletes. In both cases, by making modest changes in three external factors—activity level, meal timing, and meal composition-enormous improvements in the efficiency of their respective fitness pathways took place as measured by increased lean body mass, faster recovery, and improved muscle strength.

Yes, a calorie is a calorie. But when we increase the efficiency of the fitness engine, we derive the same or greater benefits with less energy. The technology necessary to create a green society still has to be developed, whereas the advanced metabolic technology that runs our fitness engine already has the capability to operate in an ultra-efficient manner. All we have to do is optimize the operating environment.

WHY BMI IS NOT A GOOD INDICATOR OF FITNESS

Before there was a BMI formula, health professionals used height-weight tables to determine weight status. BMI, short for body mass index, came into popular use in the 1980s. It represents a more accurate measurement of weight status for the vast majority of the population. However, BMI can be inaccurate for people who have a higher percentage of lean body mass. Since muscle weighs more than fat, people with highly developed musculature, such as athletes, have higher BMIs and are often classified as overweight by the standard BMI tables. Additionally, BMI values tend to be inaccurate for tall people and for older people who have lost significant muscle mass.

BMI classifies people into five different categories. Each category has a specific cutoff figure as shown in Table 1.1 (see next page). The cutoff figures were established by assessing the weight of thousands of individuals and establishing definitions for what constitutes normal weight, overweight, and obese. The cutoff values for BMI classifications have been modified over the years. Table 1.1 represents the latest revision.

Table 1.1. BMI Classification	
Weight Level	BMI Range
Underweight	Less than 18.5
Normal weight	18.5–24.9
Overweight	25.0–29.9
Obese	30.0–35.0
Morbidly obese	Greater than 35.0

There is little dispute that the significant increase in BMI over the years has been paralleled by an increase in people who fail to meet the minimum standards for fitness. The problem in making BMI a surrogate to define fitness is that it leads us down a path in which we fail to address the true problem. In spite of the wide availability of weight-loss products and a popular media that offers a new solution every day, the average BMI of adults (and now even children) continues to increase. Furthermore, as you will see, a focus on reducing BMI rather than on improving fitness activates adaptations within our DNA that almost guarantee that any long-term weight loss effort will fail.

Although DNA contains thousands of genes, scientists have not identified a single one whose primary action causes weight loss. At one time in human evolution, we probably possessed a mechanism that prevented excessive increases in weight since that would have made us far more susceptible to prey. Therefore, our Paleolithic ancestors had two different genes: one to efficiently store fat when there was a scarcity of food, and one to prevent obesity that would have compromised our ability to survive. There were a number of changes, however, that occurred over a million years ago that reduced or eliminated our susceptibility to predators. This included the discovery of fire, the formation of tribes, and the development of weapons. These changes would have rendered our obesity-prevention gene less useful, and ultimately, we would have lost it.

The same is not true for the genetic adaptations that enable us to efficiently store excess food as fat. For the first million years of man's evolution, the challenge was to get sufficient food to stay alive. For our ancestors, the supply of food was erratic. As a result, we developed a highly efficient metabolic system for fat storage whenever food was abundant.

While our ancestors became capable of defending themselves against predators using weapons, obesity would place most other species at greater risk from predators. Therefore, these species acquired a genetic adaptation to prevent excessive weight gain. This adaptation exists in a type of tissue known as brown adipose tissue. For example, when a rat overeats, biochemical pathways in brown adipose tissue are activated that increase the burning of fat through thermogenesis (heat loss). The excess fat is lost as body heat. Thus, the rat has a dual mechanism that maintains optimum weight. When food is in short supply, the rat stores it as fat tissue. When food is too plentiful as to potentially result in excessive weight gain, the fat is burned as heat through thermogenesis. When the phenomenon of brown adipose tissue was first discovered in animals, it, of course, set off a search to find similar tissue in humans. Alas, it took years to identify brown adipose tissue in the human body. Unfortunately, the amount we have appears to be of little consequence in helping us lose weight.

DIETING HAS LOWERED FITNESS LEVELS

The proposition that dieting has made us less fit may strike many people as equally outrageous as the proposition that dieting is a major contributor to obesity. However, as you learn more about the workings of the body's fitness circuitry, you will discover that there is substantial science to support both propositions. Consider the fact that fitness levels have declined even as our participation in dieting has increased. Not only have we become a nation of dieters, but we have become serial dieters as well. On average, adults in the United States have gone on two or more diets in the last 12 months. At any given time, 44 percent of adult women and 29 percent of adult men are dieting. When people lose weight, they lose a disproportionate amount of lean body mass. Expressed another way, if you focus only on BMI as a measure of fitness, the more weight you lose, the less fit you become. Throughout *Hardwired for Fitness*, you will discover how your body activates compensatory physiological mechanisms when you diet, which not only result in diet failure but actually make you less fit.

The second aspect of designating the terms "overweight" or "obese" as a surrogate for lack of fitness is that it is simply wrong. For example, in the last ten years there has been a growth in the number of people involved in swimming, running, cycling, and triathlons events. Participation last year was at one of the highest levels yet seen. If you watch any of these races, you will see a large number of participants who certainly exceed what the BMI table terms "normal" weight.

In the larger races, in addition to specific grouping by age and gender, there is often another group called Clydesdales. As the name implies, these are the supersized participants. Almost without exception, their BMIs would put them in the overweight to obese categories. When watching a Clydesdale participant competing in a grueling Ironman triathlon, which consists of a 1.5-mile swim, a 110-mile bike ride, and 26.2-mile run, only the delusional would suggest these individuals are not fit.

WHY FITNESS MUST BE THE GOAL

The media has created unrealistic goals in terms of our national weight. The desire to be thin (hence, popular) begins at an early age and continues throughout life. Since our BMI determines our weight classification, and because it is so easy to measure, it has become the central focus in the national health debate. Each year when the Centers for Disease Control and Prevention (CDC) publish the latest statistics (which always show an increase in BMI), it makes headlines. However, it is fitness that determines the richness of our lives. It is our ability to be fit that makes us vibrant, gives us energy, and improves our emotional outlook. These are not just the exaggerations of two authors who are obviously pro-fitness. There is considerable science to support this view.

Fit People Have More Energy

By definition, people who are physically fit have enough energy to address all the activities that have to be faced daily, and at the end of the day they still have some energy left for their families. Research indicates that a person's fitness status determines his or her perception of exertion as it relates to leisure time, occupation, and household activities. Increasing one's level of fitness reduces physical and mental fatigue and increases work productivity.

Fit People Live Longer

Small improvements in fitness level can pay significant dividends in terms of longevity. In a study published in the *New England Journal of Medicine*, investigators studied 6,000 men for a period of seven years. They found that fitness level was a stronger predictor of mortality than even age.

In another study published in the *Journal of the American Medical Association*, researchers from the University of South Carolina found that men and women older than 60, who had higher levels of fitness, lived longer than adults who were unfit, regardless of their BMI. In most cases, death rates for the most fit were 50 percent lower than the less fit.

A third study not only confirmed the previous two, but extended the conclusions. The researchers found that in men a low fitness level was associated with higher mortality risk more strongly than established risk markers, such as smoking, hypertension, diabetes, or a history of heart failure. They found that a 1,000-calorie per week increase in activity (equivalent to a 175-pound person walking about 20 minutes per day) could improve long-term survival by 20 percent.

Fit People Have Lower Disease Risk

Although there have been multiple studies on the beneficial impact of exercise in reducing disease risk factors, what is not generally recognized is that small increases in weekly activity can significantly reduce the risk of coronary heart disease. In an eight-year study published in the *New England Journal of Medicine*, researchers compared the effects of walking and vigorous exercise on coronary heart disease in 73,000 women between the ages of 40 and 65. At the time that the participants began the study, they were free of cardiovascular disease. Researchers found during the term of the study that there was a 40 percent reduction in coronary heart disease associated with both brisk walking and vigorous exercise. In other words, the women in this study received the same benefits from walking as those who engaged in vigorous exercise. The benefits derived from fitness are not just limited to cardiovascular disease. Fit people have a lower risk of developing type 2 diabetes as well as breast and colon cancer.

Fit People Have Less Anxiety and Depression

In addition to a proven effect on longevity and disease risk, fitness provides positive benefits in terms of emotional well-being. Multiple studies have correlated small increases in activity (burning 700 to 1,000 calories per week) with a significant reduction in depression. In 2000, a study involving 3,403 participants concluded that people who are fit, as measured by exercise frequency, have significantly less depression, anger, and stress than those who exercise less frequently or not at all.

Fit People Have a More Positive Attitude

Studies have consistently shown that mild increases in activity and improvement in fitness can have a profound positive effect on quality-of-life factors such as self-esteem, mood, mental stamina, and energy level. This should not be surprising, since much has been written about the mind-body connection. Most of us know that our mental state can profoundly influence our physical well-being, but what is often ignored is that our physical state can profoundly influence our mental well-being.

WHAT MAKES US FIT?

Our fitness level is determined by a composite of three factors: (1) weight or BMI, (2) body composition or percentage of body fat, and (3) activity capacity—the ability to function normally without fatigue and still be able to respond appropriately when a higher burst of energy is needed (see Figure 1.1).

When people personally describe their fitness level, they usually focus on just one of the

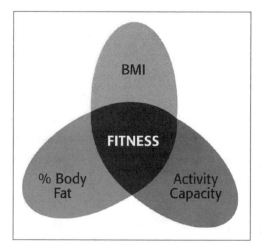

Figure 1.1. The fitness triad.

components. This translates into, "I just need to lose a few pounds," or "I have to get rid of these love handles," or "I get out of breath walking up steps." Because we are not genetically identical, each of the three components has a normal range and is influenced by our gender, our age, and, most important, our DNA.

Fortunately, all three of the essential components that determine our fitness level can be measured with a high degree of accuracy. Using these measurements, research scientists have been able to establish norms for each component.

BMI

With a few exceptions (previously noted), BMI is an accurate determination of our weight status. The normal values for BMI are shown in Table 1.2. The wide range of BMI values constituting normal weight translates into a person who is 5 feet 8 inches tall with a weight that ranges between 125 and 158 pounds. In other words, the BMI table allows considerable latitude before a person is classified as overweight.

Table 1.2. Normal BMI

Classification	Low Cut-off Point	High Cut-off Point
Normal Range	18.5	24.9

Percentage of Body Fat

Percentage of body fat is the second essential component in the fitness equation. Knowing our body fat percentage enables us to determine the amount of muscle, or lean mass we possess. The higher our fat mass, the less fit we are. Table 1.3 on the following page shows the normal ranges for the percentage of body fat of men and women.

The most accurate way to measure your percentage of body fat is in an exercise physiology laboratory; however, a number of inexpensive devices have recently been introduced to the market that make this calculation for you. Unlike BMI, which only requires us to know our height and our weight, determination of our fat percentage requires additional measurements. As

Table 1.3. Normal Ranges of Body Fat Percentage by Gender and Fitness

Classification	Women (% Fat)	Men (% Fat)
Athletes	14–20%	6–13%
Fit Individuals	21–24%	14–17%
Normal Range	25–31%	18–25%

a result, in any general discussion of obesity and fitness, percentage of body fat does not often play a prominent role—but it should. The percentage of body fat is extremely important in determining our overall level of fitness. In Part Two of this book, you will learn how to compute your body fat percentage using a simple equation.

While the percentage of body fat number tells us how much body fat we have, where this fat is located determines if we are at greater risk for specific diseases such as diabetes. The body has two types of fat: visceral fat, which is found around the abdominal cavity, and subcutaneous fat, which is the "pinchable" fat around the stomach. Aesthetically, subcutaneous fat is the more objectionable and tends to be the most difficult to lose. However, visceral fat represents a far greater health risk.

Accumulation of visceral fat results in an increase in waist size. An excess of visceral fat is known as central obesity—think potbelly or beer belly. People who have central obesity are considered apple-shaped, as opposed to pear-shaped, in which fat is deposited on the hips and buttocks. Visceral fat is associated with a higher risk of heart disease, hypertension, and type 2 diabetes.

The importance of including body fat in the fitness equation, rather than relying on BMI as the only measure of fitness, is best illustrated by a study conducted at the Mayo Clinic. Researchers measured the percentage of body fat in over 2,000 adults who had a BMI in the normal range. They found that 20 percent of the male subjects and 30 percent of the female subjects had higher body fat percentages than normal, and that these people were at greater risk for diabetes and heart disease than their peers with similar BMIs who had normal percentages of body fat. The researchers concluded that to solely focus on achieving a healthy weight or BMI in the normal range is misleading. Lean people can have an unhealthy level of body fat and be at risk for life-threatening diseases.

You will see in Chapter 4 how dieting causes an increase in body fat. Most people who diet do so because of a desire to lose body fat, but a major unintended consequence of dieting, particularly crash dieting where significant amounts of weight are lost in short periods of time, is that more than 40 percent of the total weight loss is muscle and not fat.

Activity Capacity

The third component in the fitness triad is activity capacity. Activity capacity enables us to perform day-to-day activities without fatigue and allows us to respond to situations that require a rapid expenditure of energy without undue stress. Activity capacity is also termed aerobic capacity.

Activity capacity is usually measured in a laboratory, where a person either runs on a treadmill or pedals on an exercise bike while his or her heart rate and oxygen consumption are measured simultaneously. The point at which oxygen consumption reaches a plateau as work intensity increases is the measure of a person's activity, or aerobic capacity: the higher the oxygen consumption, the greater one's activity capacity. As might be expected, activity capacity for most people declines with age, and there are also gender differences. Table 1.4 illustrates normal activity capacity in millimeters of oxygen per kilogram of body weight per minute (VO_2/kg/min) for women and between the ages of 30 and 39.

In Part Two, you will learn how to measure your own activity capacity with a fairly simple calculation following a brisk walk.

Table 1.4. Ranges of Fitness Level by Gender (Rockport Test)

Fitness Level	Women	Men
Low Fit	> 28.7	> 35.3
Moderately Fit	28.7–34.6	35.3–42.4
High Fit	34.7+	42.5+

YOU CAN BE FIT AND HAVE AN ABOVE NORMAL BMI

Your fitness level is the sum of your BMI, percentage of body fat, and activity capacity values. Because fitness is a cumulative value, your BMI value could be high, but as long as your percentage of body fat is low and your activity capacity places you in the highly fit classification, you could still be very fit. We see this in many of the Clydesdale triathlon participants, or for that matter, in many elite athletes.

A number of important studies have reinforced the value of fitness over BMI. In 1999, Dr. Steven Blair, a prominent researcher in this area, and his colleagues published a study involving more than 26,000 men. They showed a far stronger relationship between mortality and level of fitness than between mortality and BMI. In 2004, these same investigators published a study showing that fitness was a more important factor than smoking, hypertension, or diabetes as a predictor of mortality. In spite of the persuasiveness of these studies, they have had little impact on the substance of our national debate, which is still primarily about weight loss and lowering BMI.

SUMMARY

Weight is not a surrogate for fitness. Focusing on weight rather than fitness results in an overemphasis on calorie consumption rather than on improving the efficiency of the metabolic machinery that determines your level of fitness. Research strongly suggests that the obsession with dieting has actually led to an overall decrease in the fitness level of our population. Fitness is a composite of three key factors: BMI, body composition, and activity capacity. Moreover, people with BMIs in the high range can still be fit and enjoy the many benefits that fitness brings. Study after study has shown that fit people live longer, have lower disease risk, experience less anxiety and depression, and have a more positive mental attitude about life.

CHAPTER 2

Circuits and Rhythms

Long-term and permanent weight loss can only be achieved when we create the proper environment through good nutrition and daily physical activity to permit our fitness circuits to function in the manner in which they were designed. There are four circuits programmed into our DNA that determine our level of fitness. They are the (1) energy circuit, (2) appetite circuit, (3) protein turnover circuit, and (4) stress circuit. The collective action of these four circuits determines whether we have a BMI of 24 or 30, a body fat percentage of 17 or 25, or can walk a mile at a vigorous pace without our heart racing.

The body's four fitness circuits and the interrelationship between them were first described by exercise scientists, physiologists, and biochemists decades ago. Logically, you would expect energy expenditure to be closely linked to energy consumption. People who perform physical labor must consume more calories per day. A lumberjack can typically consume up to 6,000 calories per day and not gain weight. A Tour de France racer burns 6,000 calories per stage, which is why every Tour de France team has cyclists who shuttle food between the team truck and the star racer.

The fitness circuits, particularly the energy and appetite ones, are responsible for maintaining a balance between food intake and energy expenditure. What many people fail to realize is just how sophisticated this circuitry is to maintain a balance over a wide range of eating and activity behaviors. For example, the average American adult consumes a little more than a million calories a year. Data from the Centers for Disease Control and Prevention (CDC) indicate that the average American is gaining weight at the rate of one pound per year. Since a pound is equal to 3,500 calories, this means that the energy and appetite circuits, working together, are maintaining an energy balance of plus or minus 0.3 percent. Few machines can operate for years and maintain this performance tolerance. Unfortunately, that 0.3 percent imbalance between calories consumed and energy expended over the course of 30 years can dramatically change your percentage of body fat and move your BMI from a normal range into the overweight range.

To understand how to take advantage of your hardwiring, you first have to understand how the fitness circuitry works. Once you recognize the interrelationships between the circuits and how they are turned on and off, you can implement a program so that your fitness circuitry is helping you achieve your fitness goals rather than serving as an obstacle.

MASTER SWITCHES

One of the most exciting discoveries in the last decade has been the identification of molecules that have the ability to turn on specific metabolic pathways. These are the body's master switches. Each of the four fitness circuits is controlled by one—and sometimes two—master switches. When these master switches are turned on, they activate a specific sequence or circuit of metabolic reactions. The power that resides within each of the fitness circuits can only be realized when a master switch is turned on. The major master switches and the circuits they control are shown in Figure 2.1.

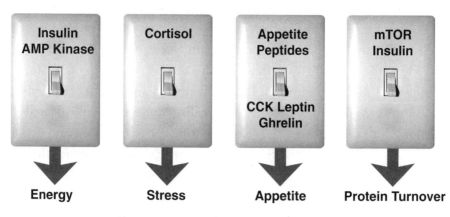

Figure 2.1. Master switches and fitness circuits.

The master switches are unique in that they are highly sensitive to a variety of internal and external stimuli. The best analogy for the master switches is the smart technology that is incorporated into modern heating systems. A computer receives information from a number of sensors that monitor outside temperature, number of people in a room, heat from lights, and humidity in the air. The smart technology collects this information and makes the appropriate adjustments in the heating, cooling, and humidity circuits.

When the master switches are turned on, they can unleash an incredible array of metabolic power. For example, activation of the protein turnover master switch has the potential to increase muscle protein synthesis or lean body mass, by more than 300 percent. When the master switch that controls appetite is turned off, it can decrease food consumption by 30 percent. When the stress master switch is turned on, hunger can increase almost threefold. When the master switch that controls the energy circuit is turned on, it can generate up to 14,400 molecules of adenosine triphosphate (ATP) per hour. ATP, the primary energy currency of the cell, provides the energy necessary to drive all metabolic reactions.

Unfortunately our modern lifestyle—including our physical activities and eating patterns—have disconnected or overloaded the fitness circuitry so that it no longer operates the way it should. The good news is this disconnection does not have to be permanent. Once reconnected, the circuits are formidable tools to help us attain our fitness goals.

Understanding how your circuitry works and creating an environment in which it can function optimally is fairly easy to do. Weight loss will no longer be a struggle. It will occur naturally as your body's fitness circuits begin to function the way in which they were designed. And the best part is not only will you be losing weight, but you will also be improving your body composition and your capacity to be active. For the first time in your life, you'll be rolling the boulder downhill!

ENERGY CIRCUIT

The energy circuit is responsible for converting the food we eat into immediate and stored energy. If the energy circuit senses that the body needs immediate energy for movement or to respond to an emergency, it converts the food, through a series of metabolic pathways, into molecules of ATP. ATP provides the energy that enables the muscles to contract, thereby providing movement. Interestingly, the body does not store a great deal of ATP. In fact, the body stores only enough ATP for a few seconds' worth of physical activity. Since the ATP storage capacity is limited, the body has developed sophisticated mechanisms to store energy, which are detailed in "How the Body Stores Energy" on page 31.

Overall, the energy circuit is remarkably efficient. From one molecule of simple sugar, the muscles can create 36 molecules of ATP, and from one triglyceride molecule, the muscles can create 460 molecules of ATP.

Energy Circuit Master Switches

The two master switches that control the energy circuit are an enzyme called AMP kinase and the hormone insulin. AMP kinase is the energy sensor for cells. Muscle cells are somewhat unique in that their demand for energy can rise a hundredfold in a minute's notice. When AMP kinase detects a rapid decline in ATP stores, it turns on the energy circuit to ensure the cells' energy needs are maintained. This includes activating the cellular machinery for the conversion of fat into energy and the transport of sugar into muscle, where it is converted into ATP to drive muscle contraction.

The second energy master switch is insulin. According to much of the popular media and well-known diet books, insulin is the cause of obesity in our society. Hundreds of millions of dollars have been made by developing diet plans and products around a theme of insulin bashing. This obsession with insulin has also resulted in diet recommendations that are unhealthy over the long-term and make it all but impossible to keep weight off and achieve the level of fitness most people desire.

Functionally, insulin, which is produced by the pancreas, is one of the most important master switches in the body. It plays a central role in energy regulation by transporting simple sugars into the cell where they are converted into energy for muscle movement as well as controlling many other critical functions related to tissue repair and growth. When energy

How the Body Stores Energy

The energy circuit converts most of our food into stored energy. Energy is stored as one of three forms. The first form of stored energy is creatine phosphate (CP). CP represents the most rapid form of stored fuel for replenishing ATP. There is a sufficient amount of CP stored in the muscle to support a maximal effort for 8 to 12 seconds, but without this system, fast, powerful movements such as sprinting or weight lifting could not be performed. Of course, CP must be replenished rapidly to help support the replenishment of ATP during physical activity. For this, we have other fuel sources that are stored in much greater concentrations.

The second form of energy stored is glycogen, which is abundantly stockpiled in muscle and in the liver. Glycogen is simply a complex of glucose molecules. For it to be used, it must first be broken down into glucose, a simple sugar. The energy released from the breakdown of muscle glycogen can be used to provide rapid replenishment of ATP directly or indirectly via the replenishment of CP. The glycogen stored in the liver is used to maintain normal levels of glucose in the blood. During exercise, blood glucose becomes a very important source of energy for contracting muscles. When the muscles use blood glucose faster than the liver can resupply it, hypoglycemia (low blood sugar) results and fatigue ensues.

The third form of stored energy is fat. Fat is mainly stored in adipose tissue as triglycerides, but triglycerides are also stored in muscle cells. Stored fat or triglycerides come mainly from the fat in our diet. However, carbohydrate can be converted into fat when our storage limit for carbohydrate has been met. Fat is a very efficient way to store energy. One gram of fat provides more than twice as much energy as one gram of carbohydrate. Fat stored in adipose tissue is not readily available for use by the muscle. First it must be broken down into free fatty acids and then transported via the blood to the muscle. Within the muscle, the free fatty acids are further broken down, releasing energy for the production of ATP. This is not a very fast process; therefore, energy from free fatty acids can be used only during low-to-moderate intensity exercise or physical activity. While fat utilization can be rather slow, the ability to store fat, much to our dismay, is a very efficient mechanism.

demands are low, insulin plays a key role in storing the food we eat into muscle and liver glycogen and fat in the form of triglycerides.

AMP kinase and insulin work in opposition to each other. AMP kinase increases the utilization of fuel sources when energy demands are high, and insulin increases the storage of fuel sources when energy demands are low.

Energy Circuit Timing

We are not nocturnal creatures. We are programmed by our circadian clock to expend most of our energy during daylight hours. Logic would therefore dictate that the energy circuit responsible for balancing energy consumption and energy needs would be most active during the day, and that is, indeed, what occurs, as shown in Figure 2.2. In the evening, overall activity of the energy circuit diminishes, reaching a low while we are sleeping.

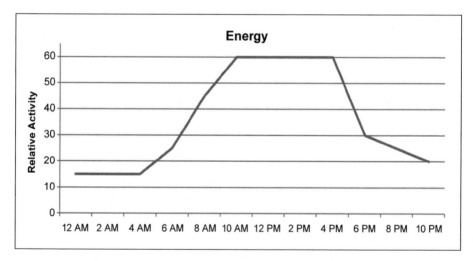

Figure 2.2. Natural metabolic rhythm of the energy circuit.

APPETITE CIRCUIT

Appetite is the second key circuit that helps define our level of fitness. Our desire to eat ensures that we consume adequate amounts of food to provide the energy we need to survive on a daily basis. Appetite is regulated by interactions of the brain, digestive tract, and adipose tissue through the release of hormones and small proteins or peptides and neurotransmitters. There are actually two parts to the appetite circuit. One part involves sensing hunger, which is controlled by the hypothalamus. The hypothalamus is a portion of the brain that controls many critical functions such as sleep and body temperature. When our bodies are deprived of food for extended periods, the hunger sensors are activated, the appetite center in the brain is stimulated, and we seek out food. Once we find food, we eat until we become full, and then another group of sensors are activated that stimulate the satiety center of the brain. This tells us to stop eating.

For the first million years of our existence, food was generally in short supply. Therefore, it should not be surprising that we have more sensors that turn on appetite than turn off appetite. When food was available, our Paleolithic ancestors continued to eat, and their very efficient energy circuit converted the excess food into fat. When food was scarce, fat stores could be easily mobilized to provide the needed energy to permit our Paleolithic ancestors to function and survive until a new source of food was found.

Appetite Circuit Master Switches

There are two types of master switches that control appetite. One switch responds to hunger. This switch, as you might expect, is closely linked to the master switches that control energy. When the body senses that its energy levels are low, the hunger master switch, ghrelin, a small hormone released by the cells of the stomach, signals the brain to tell us to start eating. Ghrelin turns on appetite by activating sensors in the hunger center of the brain, the hypothalamus.

The fullness master switch, cholecystokinin (CCK), a small protein found primarily in cells in the small intestine, tells us to stop eating. CCK responds to signals in the stomach. CCK works by closing down the valve that leads from the stomach into the intestines. In doing so, food cannot move as quickly from the stomach into the gastrointestinal tract. As the food builds up in the stomach, it expands and we become quite uncomfortable. At the same time, CCK sends a signal to the brain that tells us to stop eating.

If the hardwiring that controls these two switches had evolved in the environment that exists in the United States today where food is plentiful, it would have been programmed very differently. The fullness switch would be far more sensitive. Unfortunately, this environment did not exist for our Paleolithic ancestors. Therefore, the mechanisms that turn on appetite are far more developed than the mechanisms that turn off appetite.

Appetite Circuit Timing

Similar to the energy circuit, the appetite circuit has a specific biological rhythm. Figure 2.3 illustrates the metabolic rhythm of the hunger pathway. It is low late at night and in the early morning hours and increases in late morning, mid-afternoon, and evening.

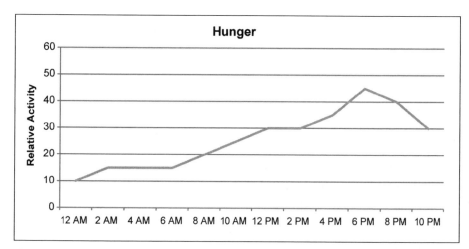

Figure 2.3. Natural metabolic rhythm of the hunger pathway of the appetite circuit.

PROTEIN TURNOVER CIRCUIT

The protein turnover circuit controls protein levels in the body. The protein turnover circuit consists of two pathways. One pathway manufactures (synthesizes) proteins and the other pathway breaks down (degrades) proteins. Throughout the day, proteins are constantly being made and broken down. This dynamic process is called protein turnover. When protein turnover favors synthesis, protein accumulation occurs, and the body increases lean body mass. When protein turnover favors degradation, the body loses lean body mass.

Although fat and carbohydrate are critical for health and well-being, protein has a special place in the hierarchy of nutrients. Proteins are used to make up cell structure, form enzymes, and even provide fuel for energy-requiring processes. Enzymes are the molecules that mediate the tens of thousands of biochemical reactions that take place in our cells every minute. For example, although carbohydrate and fat are critical sources of energy, it is protein, via enzymes, that enables the body to convert carbohydrate and fat to ATP. Because proteins make up the major structural molecules of the cell, it is the primary measurement of lean body mass. About 65 percent of the body's protein stores are found in our muscles.

The protein that makes up cell structures and enzymes is constantly turning over. That is, it is regularly being replaced with new protein. This is a very important process, because it ensures that damaged protein is efficiently replaced. As we age, however, the rate of protein turnover declines, and if we don't take the proper steps we lose lean body mass.

When more protein is broken down than is being made, the body is in a negative protein balance, or a catabolic state. This occurs in many wasting diseases, such as cancer or AIDS. When more protein is being manufactured than is being broken down, the body is in a positive protein balance, or an anabolic state. An anabolic state is required for building lean body mass. This anabolic state generally follows an increase in physical activity, as long as the body's nutritional needs are satisfied.

Under most circumstances during a 24-hour interval, the body is in protein balance (neither positive nor negative). However, during specific segments of the day, it may be out of balance. For example, late at night or in the early morning hours, the body tends to be in negative protein balance; during the day, in protein balance; and in the evening, in positive protein balance.

Protein Turnover Circuit Master Switches

The protein turnover circuit has two master switches, mTOR and insulin (yes, insulin again). The mTOR switch is a protein found in all cells, from the muscle to the brain. Its primary function is to activate the metabolic pathways that synthesize new protein needed as a result of normal growth or physical activity, or protein damaged due to the body's normal physiological functions.

You probably thought insulin was only involved in carbohydrate metabolism. However, insulin also plays a primary role in building muscle protein by helping transport the building blocks of protein—amino acids—into the cell, where they can be linked together to form enzymes and structural proteins that are essential for life. Insulin also reduces protein breakdown. Insulin can increase lean body mass three ways: (1) it activates mTOR, which stimulates protein synthesis, (2) it stimulates protein synthesis independently of mTOR, and (3) it slows the breakdown of protein. Remember, lean body mass is the net result of both protein synthesis and protein breakdown.

Protein Turnover Circuit Timing

The body's number-one metabolic priority is to supply energy to drive all of its biochemical reactions, as well as to supply energy for muscle activity. Anytime there is a competing metabolic need such as synthesis of new protein, energy production wins out. Since rebuilding protein requires energy, it is logical that the activity of the protein turnover circuit is low during the day when muscle energy needs are greatest. This is shown in Figure 2.4, which illustrates the natural metabolic rhythm of the protein turnover circuit. When energy needs begin to diminish, the protein turnover circuit becomes far more active, particularly in the early evening. The hours between 5:00 P.M. and 8:00 P.M. represent the optimal time to increase protein synthesis, thereby building lean body mass. In the early morning hours, while we are sleeping, the protein degradation pathway is turned on to insure that the body has the necessary energy to maintain baseline function.

The natural metabolic rhythm of the protein turnover circuit also illustrates the fallacy of consuming a high-protein/low-carbohydrate diet during the day, the time when energy needs are highest. On this type of diet, protein becomes a primary source for energy rather than for building lean

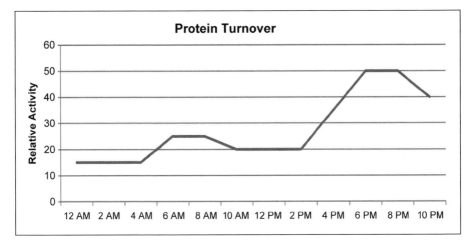

Figure 2.4. Natural metabolic rhythm of the protein turnover circuit.

mass. The breakdown of protein is much less efficient at producing ATP than carbohydrate. That's why people on high-protein/low-carbohydrate diets often feel tired and lack energy.

STRESS CIRCUIT

Stress is defined as an external force that interferes with the normal physiological functions of the body. The problem with this definition is it fails to take into account that stress is also a natural internal force that maintains normal physiological functions. In any discussion of fitness, the differences between physical and psychological stress must be recognized. Modern society is characterized by high levels of psychological stress. Sustained levels of psychological stress have been shown to be a primary risk factor of cardiovascular disease, type 2 diabetes, cancer, and mental disorders. Physical stress, on the other hand, is not only a critical part of our survival mechanism but it also plays an important role in the efficient functioning of the body's fitness circuitry. Almost everyone is familiar with the body's "fight-or-flight response"—its stress-response system. In the presence of immediate danger, the stress circuit is activated, mobilizing specific pathways that provide the muscles with the necessary energy to get out of danger. The stress circuit also lowers the body's sensitivity to pain, and increases immunity to disease. When you work out, stress gives your muscles the additional push and your brain the mental toughness to do one more rep or run one more mile.

Stress represents a vital circuit in helping us maintain fitness. Normally, the stress circuit is activated quickly and then turned off following a stressful event. The stress circuit is also activated during periods of calorie restriction. When the stress circuit is turned on, it activates the metabolic pathways responsible for breaking down fat and protein so that the body has a consistent supply of energy, even when we are sleeping. On the negative side, persistent stress can have adverse emotional, physiological, and metabolic consequences. High levels of unresolved stress can negatively impact normal functioning of the energy, appetite, and protein turnover circuits.

Stress Circuit Master Switch

The hormone cortisol is the master switch that turns on the stress circuit. Among supplement manufacturers, cortisol has replaced insulin as the culprit that causes obesity. Their reasoning is that when cortisol levels are perpetually elevated, it increases hunger and also increases abdominal fat. Although this is true, even if cortisol-lowering supplements worked—which they don't—they would not address the problem of being overweight.

From a physiological perspective, stress is a critical survival mechanism. At times when energy levels fall, cortisol stimulates the breakdown of fat and protein so that they can be efficiently used as energy. Remember, fat is the most efficient way the body can store energy. When the body requires a significant but short-term amount of energy, a rise in cortisol in the blood is one of the mechanisms that provide it. Obviously, cortisol has its place in regulating energy metabolism. However, when cortisol is perpetually elevated, it can lead to overeating, increased body fat, metabolic disorders, and cardiovascular problems.

Stress Circuit Timing

The stress circuit is activated by both psychological and physiological stressors. Psychological stress can occur anytime, especially in modern society.

Physiological stress, however, has its own circadian rhythm, as shown in Figure 2.5.

The natural metabolic pattern of the stress circuit reflects the circadian adaptations within our DNA. The late evening and early morning hours represent the longest period of the day that the body goes without food. To meet its resting energy requirements, cortisol stimulates the pathways that break down fat and protein for energy. This provides sufficient energy to get us through the night.

Cortisol also stimulates the hunger master switch ghrelin. After an eight-hour fast, ghrelin's function is to tell the brain that the body has to be fed. During the day, cortisol levels are low due to physiological conditions, but that may not hold true for psychological stress. Psychological stress can occur at any time, resulting in an increase in cortisol levels. The stress response can disrupt the normal functioning of the body's metabolic rhythm. It is difficult to eliminate psychological stress from our lives. However, as you will learn, you can take specific steps to reduce stress.

WHY TIMING IS SO CRITICAL

Turning on the four fitness circuits without regard to function would create metabolic chaos, because actions of certain circuits may be in conflict

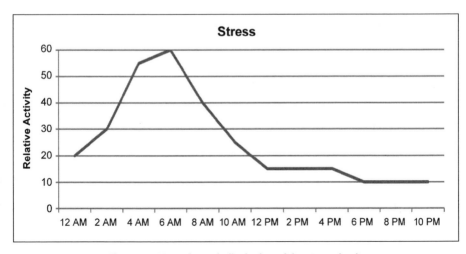

Figure 2.5. Natural metabolic rhythm of the stress circuit.

with others. For example, turning off hunger would not be beneficial following a period in which muscle energy stores were depleted. In order to prevent this from happening, the four circuits are in constant communication with each other. This is a very sophisticated and integrated communication network, as you will learn in next chapter.

SUMMARY

Four specific highly integrated circuits—energy, appetite, stress, and protein turnover—determine your overall level of fitness. Researchers in the last ten years have identified the link between these circuits as well as the master switches that control them. One of the most important discoveries is that each of these circuits has a unique natural metabolic rhythm. By synchronizing both when you eat and what you eat to these natural metabolic rhythms, you unleash a powerful tool that enables you to achieve your long-term fitness goals. Instead of fighting your body, making minor changes in your lifestyle activity levels and diet can optimize the functioning of your fitness circuitry.

CHAPTER 3

High-Speed Communication Network

Each of the body's four fitness circuits is an amazing stand-alone metabolic engine. Take the energy circuit, for example. The energy circuit has the capacity to produce as much as 10,000 calories of energy per day or as few as 1,500 calories per day, and still maintain its high level of efficiency. After intense physical activity, in which muscle energy stores are depleted, the energy circuit can replenish them in as little as six hours. Additionally, the energy circuit has sensors that allow it to adjust rapidly to changes in the operating environment.

An automobile engine is similar to the body's energy circuit in that both convert fuel into energy plus heat. The efficiency of a car engine is measured by how much energy it produces. Most automobile engines are about 19 percent efficient. For each gallon of fuel consumed, the engine converts 19 percent into energy and the remaining 81 percent as heat. If the heat is not quickly removed through the cooling system, the engine will seize up.

The body's energy circuit is almost 50 percent more efficient than a car engine. In spite of this increased efficiency, 72 percent of the food we consume is lost as heat. This helps maintain body temperature. During high muscle activity, the amount of heat generated increases geometrically. Without a cooling mechanism, 25 minutes of intense exercise would increase the body's temperature to 105°F, which is close to the lethal range. To prevent this, the energy circuit removes the heat building up in the muscle by increasing the flow of blood from the muscles to the skin. The increased heat is released in the form of sweat, which has a cooling effect.

The cooled blood then returns to the muscles to continue the heat removal cycle.

The energy circuit is also extremely adaptable. It can convert all three macronutrients—carbohydrates, fats, and proteins—into energy. Although it has this capacity, the energy utilization pathway does not treat all three macronutrients equally. There is a metabolic priority system. For short bursts of energy, carbohydrate is the preferred macronutrient. For longer-term activity, fat becomes a major source of energy. For extended periods of activity, the energy circuit begins to break down protein. The "sparing" effect of protein represents an important adaptation. Since our Paleolithic ancestors did not know when they would be consuming protein, and since protein is so critical for body structure, the energy circuit conserves protein, only using it when it is necessary.

The other three fitness circuits are equally exceptional. The appetite circuit has the ability to sense how much energy is stored in muscle and fat, and responds accordingly. It also has a high level of redundancy. Because consumption of food is critical to survival, if we only had one pathway that controlled food intake, the result would have been catastrophic for our species if for some reason it failed to function. To ensure this would never happen, the appetite circuit has elements in the gastrointestinal tract, brain, and adipose tissue that can monitor and provide the stimulus that encourages us to eat when fuel stores are low.

The protein turnover circuit is responsible for maintaining muscle mass, which includes its repair, rebuilding, and development. Locomotion is an essential factor in the ability to survive. That's why muscle makes up as much as 50 percent of the total weight of body tissue. The protein turnover circuit can manufacture from 20 to 40 grams of protein per day during resistance exercise training. This would amount to an increase of four to five pounds of muscle in 10 weeks of training.

Similarly, the stress circuit has the capacity to mobilize any and all nutrients stored in the body for energy when confronted with a life-threatening situation. The reaction time for the stress circuit is measured in seconds. When food is in short supply, the stress circuit can manipulate multiple pathways to ensure that the critical life-maintaining processes have the energy necessary to continue functioning.

CIRCUITRY INTEGRATION

The most amazing attribute of the body's fitness circuits, however, is their ability to communicate and act in a coordinated fashion. Through multiple cross connections, the circuits are linked to each other as shown in Figure 3.1. Circuitry integration is the primary reason why your body has the ability to respond to many different environmental stimuli. Since the function of one circuit could metabolically cancel out the effect of another, the lack of a coordinated control would create physiological anarchy. Think of a sophisticated heating and air conditioning system that was not controlled by a common thermostat. You could have both heating and air conditioning units working at the same time. Imagine what would happen if your appetite circuit was not connected to your energy circuit. You could potentially deplete your energy stores without a hunger signal telling you to seek out and consume more food.

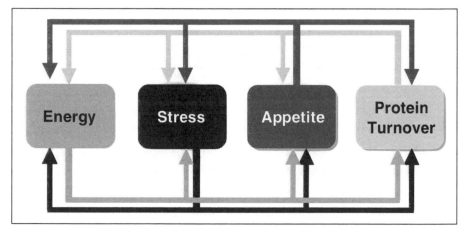

Figure 3.1. Circuitry integration.

The tight integration between the four fitness circuits is responsible, in large part, for the body's ability to respond quickly and efficiently to a wide range of both positive and negative situations and to restore normal physiological balance. Integration and communication among the four fitness circuits gives the system the capability to operate at high levels for extended periods of time, troubleshoot and correct problems, and work efficiently in almost every conceivable situation and environment. Circuitry integration also explains, as you shall see, why the singular approach of almost all diets and fitness programs is predestined to fail over time.

The heart of circuitry integration is the master switches (discussed in Chapter 2). Think of the master switches as the body's control boxes. The master switches constantly receive information from the many sensors that monitor the body's internal and external environments. Although all the subtleties of the system aren't understood, we do know that the master switches are hardwired to each other. The best way to illustrate this coordination is to look at how the circuits respond to different situations. Circuitry integration also is best understood if you never lose sight of the fact that the overriding priority of the fitness circuitry is to insure that the processes critical for survival always have sufficient energy to function.

Sustained Moderate-to-High Energy Expenditure

Sustained moderate-to-high energy expenditure commonly occurs during exercise such as running a 5-kilometer race or skiing, or during a daily activity such as raking leaves or shoveling snow.

Figure 3.2 illustrates that during exercise the need for energy to drive muscle contraction is the highest priority. As to be expected, the energy utilization pathway is turned on while simultaneously turning the energy storage pathway off. What may not be so obvious is the effect of exercise on the appetite, protein turnover, and stress circuits.

During moderate-to-high intensity prolonged exercise, blood flow that normally supplies the gastrointestinal tract is shunted to the muscles, since they have the greatest need for oxygen. This hampers the body's ability to digest food, so it is not surprising that the hunger pathway is switched off and the pathway that controls fullness is turned on. This effect continues for several hours, which explains why exercise produces a short-term suppression of appetite.

The stress circuit remains in a standby mode as long as there are sufficient energy stores within the muscle. When muscle energy stores fall below a critical level, the stress circuit springs into action stimulating the

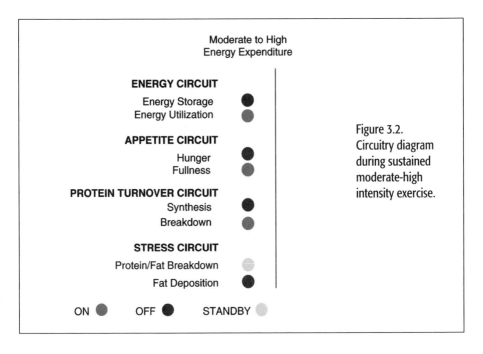

Figure 3.2. Circuitry diagram during sustained moderate-high intensity exercise.

breakdown of both fat and protein for use as energy to maintain muscle activity. Since the manufacture and repair of protein requires energy, the protein synthesis pathway is turned off. This avoids any competition for energy between the protein synthesis and energy utilization pathways. In fact, the opposite may occur. If the stress circuit determines that energy use will be extended, it turns on the protein degradation pathway. This initiates a series of biochemical reactions culminating in the use of muscle protein as an energy source.

The integration between the four fitness circuits is seamless. We are usually not aware of how our circuitry is acting in concert to ensure that our muscles have a continual supply of energy during exercise.

Food Restriction and Overeating

The two extremes of food restriction and overeating represented the norm for our Paleolithic ancestors. Food was generally in short supply and involuntary caloric restriction the norm. Following a hunt, the situation changed dramatically. Involuntary caloric restriction was followed by overeating. Today, these two diverse situations coexist. The only difference is that caloric restriction, for the most part today, is voluntary. Food, particularly energy-dense food, is abundant and cheap, and caloric restriction or dieting is an integral part of our modern lifestyle. When one compares the circuitry diagrams in these two diverse situations, some surprising observations become readily apparent (Figure 3.3).

First, let's examine what happens during calorie restriction. Sensors within the hunger center of the brain recognize there is a depletion of the body's energy stores and the hunger circuit is turned on. Simultaneously, the energy circuit dials down the energy expenditure pathway to preserve energy stores for as long as possible. A consequence of this circuitry interaction is that we feel tired and fatigue easily.

The stress circuit becomes the primary player as sensors detect an energy shortage. When the stress circuit is switched on, it institutes a number of coordinated actions. The result—the hunger pathway is activated, and fat stores and muscle protein are metabolized for energy. If the food shortage persists, the fitness circuits go into survival mode. Unfortunately, as you will see, the sensors cannot distinguish between a true food

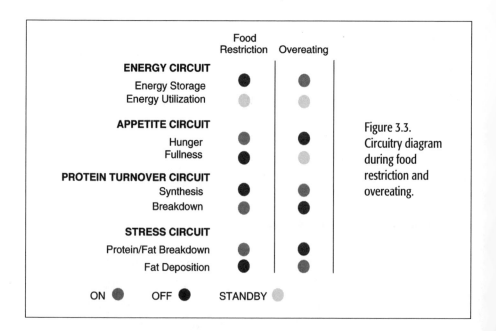

Figure 3.3. Circuitry diagram during food restriction and overeating.

shortage such as a famine and an artificially created one such as a crash diet.

During overeating, one would expect the coordinated response of the fitness circuitry to be quite different. That generally is the case. Ideally, when we overeat we would like to see the energy utilization pathway switched on to burn off the excess calories. Unfortunately, the coordinated response is to store, not burn, the excess energy. Looking at the circuit diagram for overeating, you see that the energy storage, fat deposition, and protein synthesis pathways are all switched on. Although the hunger circuit is turned off, the fullness circuit does not react quickly. Therefore, we continue to eat before having the sensation of fullness, which signals us to stop eating.

Two very different situations, which provoke very different circuit responses, yet surprisingly, both situations result in a decrease in our overall level of fitness. Food restriction decreases lean body mass as muscle protein is metabolized into energy, and stimulates our desire to eat. Overeating increases fat storage particularly abdominal fat without strongly curbing our desire to eat.

Sustained Physical and/or Psychological Stress When Food Is Abundant

Stress plays a critical role in helping us cope with extreme physiological situations. During periods of high stress, the four circuits mobilize to maximize energy production. The normal stress response is short-lived. Today, however, we have an external environment that was unanticipated by our hardwiring. We live in a very stressful world. Thus, we have high stress at the same time that energy in the form of calorically dense food is cheap and plentiful. This combination plays havoc with any attempt to lose weight and get in shape.

The circuitry diagram (Figure 3.4 on the following page) shows the impact of chronic stress. A sustained elevation of the stress hormone, cortisol, activates the hunger center of the brain increasing the desire to eat. Cortisol also promotes fat storage, particularly in the abdominal region.

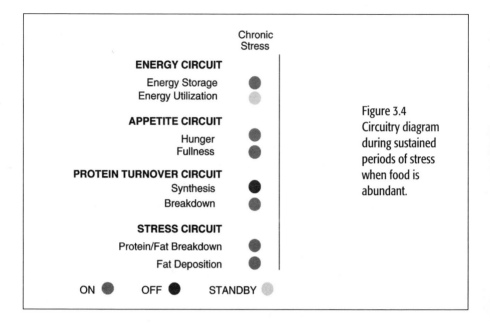

Figure 3.4 Circuitry diagram during sustained periods of stress when food is abundant.

Finally, a sustained level of cortisol can result in protein breakdown leading to a lower metabolic rate, weakened muscles, and a lower energy level.

In the presence of sustained levels of stress, circuitry integration has a detrimental impact on all three of the components that make up the fitness triad: BMI, body fat percentage, and activity capacity. It seems illogical. Why would our bodies marshal our incredible metabolic capabilities to make us less fit? How does a powerful force for fitness became an equally powerful force for unfitness? Two reasons: (1) our bodies have not adapted to living in a world characterized by high and sustained levels of stress. Our stress mechanism is designed for situational stress. (2) Our stress sensors can't tell the difference between physiological and psychological or emotional stressors.

This last reason illustrates a major defect in the fitness circuitry. The sensors that feed information to the master switches can't determine if the stimuli are natural or simulated. Is it a famine, or is it a diet? Are we running from prey, or are we going through a divorce? Have we just killed a deer for dinner, or are we attending an extended round of holiday parties?

The inability of our metabolic sensors to distinguish between real and simulated conditions is a major impediment on our path to fitness.

SUMMARY

Circuitry integration is the most amazing attribute of your fitness mechanisms. Circuitry integration enables the four circuits to respond to a wide range of internal and external factors in a coordinated fashion. The heart of circuitry integration is the master switches, which receive information from multiple sensors. Because the master switches are hardwired to each other, they can coordinate the action of each circuit to restore the body's normal physiological balance. Integration and communication among the four fitness circuits give the system the capability to operate at high levels for extended periods of time, to troubleshoot and correct problems, and to work efficiently in almost every conceivable situation and environment. Failure to recognize the critical role that circuitry integration plays in fitness is the primary reason why almost all diet and fitness programs fail over the long-term.

CHAPTER 4

Disconnected and Overloaded Circuits

Because the environment of our Paleolithic ancestors was characterized by dramatic changes, an inability of our fitness circuitry to respond would have been catastrophic. The integration and cross connections of the fitness circuits permit our bodies to respond to changes in the food supply, in the types of food we consume, and in our energy needs.

Think about a machine that engineers had the luxury of fine-tuning over 1 million years. They would have had the opportunity to troubleshoot, adjust, and tweak the machine, to install upgrades, and to reprogram and modify the operating system to ensure that it had the capacity to perform optimally, regardless of how dramatically the operating environment changed.

This describes the body's fitness circuitry. When needed, it can respond almost instantaneously, anticipate a negative change in the environment, react to a temporary overload or even a momentary disconnection, utilize a variety of different fuel sources, diagnose an operating problem, and even repair itself—and we're not talking about science fiction here!

The fitness circuitry has one other important property: if it should become temporarily out of balance, it can resynchronize itself so that it continues to operate at optimum efficiency. However, the fitness circuitry doesn't have the capacity to quickly rebalance and resynchronize itself when the operating conditions undergo a continuing change. Recognizing how adaptable this fitness circuitry is, it's hard to believe that in little more than 50 years we have changed the operating environment so significantly that the circuitry cannot adapt. The results of this circuitry overload are readily apparent by the prevalence of obesity. In spite of the fact that more Americans are exercising regularly than ever before, the segment of the population that is not exercising is becoming less fit when evaluated by the fitness triad: BMI, percentage of body fat, and activity capacity. (It is surprising that no one has yet published a study blaming exercise for the rise in obesity.)

Unfortunately, this circuit dysfunction is not caused by a single factor but rather by multiple changes in our environment, lifestyle, and nutrition choices. To reestablish the body's natural metabolic rhythm, we have to address all the following conditions:

• Not meeting the mandatory activity threshold

• Constant dieting

• Unresolved stress

• Nutrition choices that ignore changes in body function over the day

• Change in sleep patterns

• The perpetual meal (eating small meals and snacks frequently throughout the day)

Looking at each one of these factors in greater depth will help you better understand why these changes have created a dysfunctional fitness circuitry.

NOT MEETING THE MANDATORY ACTIVITY THRESHOLD

Although the fitness circuitry can perform exceedingly well over a wide range of energy needs, the circuitry requires a minimum level of activity to function properly. For the first million years of our existence, meeting the minimum level of daily activity was never a problem. Activity involved in hunting and gathering food was a prerequisite for survival. The problems only arose in the last 50 years when daily activity levels approached the minimal levels essential for proper function of the fitness circuitry.

Most obesity and fitness experts disagree on the best approach to combat the problem. However, there is a general consensus that a major cause of obesity is a more sedentary lifestyle. But, as you will see, that is only part of the reason. Studies certainly support this hypothesis. In the last five decades, we have seen dramatic increases in BMI values. These increases in BMI did not occur through changes in our DNA. Adaptations to DNA take place over hundreds of thousands and even millions of years, not 50 years. The increase in BMI has resulted from lifestyle changes that have impacted the body's fitness circuits.

In 1850, the military conducted a health survey among 12,000 retired soldiers. The average BMI for this group was 23. Only 2 percent had a BMI higher than 30. The average BMI among the American population remained relatively unchanged between 1850 and the beginning of the 20th century. In fact, as late as 1950, the average BMI was 24. Although occupational activity (that is, farming and factory jobs) declined throughout the 20th century, even in 1960 when more of our workforce was employed in white-collar jobs, daily activity was still above the minimum level to assure that the fitness circuitry worked properly.

From 1960 to 2002, the changes were astonishing. During this period, men and women on average gained 24 pounds. The average BMI increased from 25 to 28. Keep in mind that a BMI between 22 and 25 is considered normal. In 2009, the Centers for Disease Control and Prevention (CDC) reported that 66 percent of American adults were either overweight or obese.

This increase in obesity has been paralleled by an increase in sedentary activity. Active factory workers became sedentary desk workers. Reliance on the automobile and an increase in sedentary activities, such as watching television and working and playing on computers, have all contributed to the problem because more and more of our population are not expending the minimum level of calories to ensure that our fitness circuitry works as engineered. Recent studies observed that adults spent 55 to 57 percent of their waking hours in sedentary activities.

Our Bodies' Energy Use

Understanding the body's energy use is fundamental to understanding how the fitness circuits work. Normally, the circuitry works flawlessly but under certain conditions it can malfunction as discussed in this section. The total amount of energy the body requires is derived from three components: (1) resting energy expenditure, (2) thermic energy expenditure, and (3) lifestyle energy expenditure.

Resting energy expenditure refers to the amount of energy that the body needs just to stay alive. It is measured when we are resting or lying down. There are precise formulas to determine resting energy expenditure. Resting energy expenditure is a direct function of muscle or lean body mass because muscle tissue burns more calories than all the other body tissues combined. For example, a 40-year-old, 5 feet 11 inches tall, 190-pound male would have a resting energy expenditure of about 1,879 calories per day. Expressed another way, this individual would have to consume 1,879 calories each day just to maintain his weight even if he performed no physical activity. In Chapter 8, we will show you a simple method to determine your resting energy expenditure.

The second component, thermic energy expenditure, refers to the amount of calories a person burns by eating and digesting food. This represents about 6 to 8 percent of one's resting energy expenditure. A great deal of misinformation has been written about consuming meals that have a high thermic effect. Its contribution to energy expenditure is rather minor, and therefore, its impact on total daily energy expenditure is usually ignored.

Lifestyle energy expenditure is the third—and perhaps the most important—contributor to a person's total daily expenditure. This component is highly relevant to fitness and determines whether the fitness circuitry functions properly. Lifestyle energy expenditure, as you might imagine, varies greatly because it is a function of an individual's daily activity. Our Paleolithic ancestors most likely had a lifestyle energy expenditure of 3,000 calories per day. If, for example, a 190-pound man has a resting energy expenditure of 1,879 calories per day, as shown in Figure 4.1 depending on lifestyle and occupation, his total daily energy expenditure could range from 2,255 (sedentary) to 3,570 (extra active).

We are hardwired to perform a minimum level of activity per day, and once we attain that minimum level, there is a strong relationship between daily activity and caloric consumption. When we go below this level, we

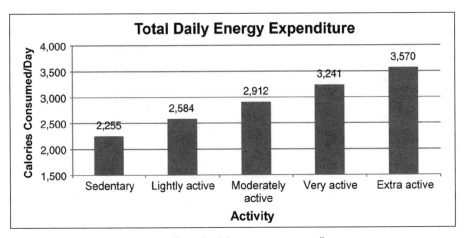

Figure 4.1. Effect of activity on energy expenditure.

disconnect the circuits that normally link appetite to energy expenditure to building lean body mass. Attaining your threshold level each day is fundamental to achieving your fitness goals.

The disconnection phenomenon was first observed in a landmark study conducted over 50 years ago by the late Dr. Jean Mayer, one of the great nutritionists of the 20th century. Dr. Mayer and his coworkers measured daily caloric expenditure among people with different occupations—ranging from clerks to laborers—that required different levels of physical activity.

As shown in Figure 4.2, Mayer found that there was a tight coupling or connection between average daily energy expenditure and calorie consumption. Individuals who had jobs (such as laborers) requiring very high-energy expenditures also had high-energy consumption. Thus, they stayed in energy balance, neither gaining nor losing weight. Dr. Mayer found that energy balance was maintained over a wide range of daily physical activities. However, when energy expenditure fell below a certain daily level (look at moderately sedentary to very sedentary individuals), the relationship between energy expenditure and calorie consumption broke down or became uncoupled. In fact, when daily energy requirements declined below a certain threshold level, calorie consumption actually increased. In other words, the least active individuals ate more than the more active counterparts. Mayer's results showed that when physical

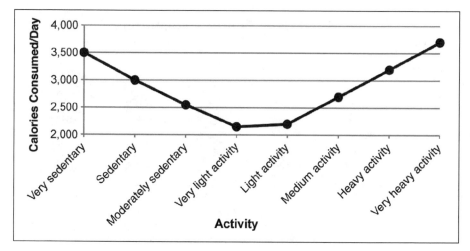

Figure 4.2. Effect of activity on calorie expenditure.

activity is reduced beyond a certain level there is an uncoupling between the energy and appetite circuits.

There is nothing breakthrough about suggesting that when we fail to meet a minimum level of activity, we gain weight because we are not converting all the food we eat to energy. However, what Mayer showed and has been ignored by the experts is that when people fail to meet a threshold level of activity the appetite circuit is overly stimulated. It is the worst of all scenarios when you're attempting to lose weight. You are not burning all the calories you are consuming and you are eating more because you feel hungry.

As expected, Dr. Mayer also saw increased weight (Figure 4.3) in individuals who were below the activity threshold, whereas the weight of those above the activity threshold remained stable, since energy intake remained proportional to energy expenditure. Mayer's work illustrates just how interconnected the appetite and energy circuits are, and why a minimum level of daily activity is an essential condition in order for the fitness circuitry to work properly. The starting point for any fitness program is not altering your calorie intake but making sure you are achieving your threshold level of activity each day.

The disconnect between the energy and appetite circuits when we go below the threshold level was further confirmed in a study by Dr. John

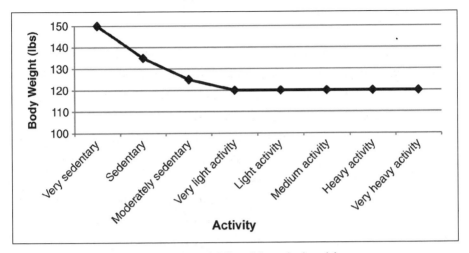

Figure 4.3. Effect of daily activity on body weight.

Blundell, one of the world's leading experts on appetite. Dr. Blundell and his coworkers measured the impact of physical activity on appetite in normal weight subjects while they were either moderately active or sedentary.

They found that when the subjects were sedentary, there was no parallel reduction in food intake. In other words, during the sedentary phase, the subjects continued to eat as much as when they were moderately active. Additionally, during the sedentary period, the subjects were more preoccupied with thoughts of food and had a greater urge to eat. During the sedentary period, *almost twice as many of the unburned calories were converted into fat*, which would have translated into a weight gain of 30 pounds over the span of 12 months.

Survey data over the past 200 years provide strong support that an increase in sedentary lifestyle is one of the prime reasons for an increase in BMI and a decrease in fitness level. However, much of the prevailing wisdom simply looks at exercise in terms of the first law of thermodynamics—the more a person exercises, the more calories he or she burns. What has not been recognized is that the body requires a minimum or threshold level of activity every day in order for the fitness circuits to function properly. The good news is the research also shows that lifestyle activity plays a far more important role than exercise. In Chapter 8, you will learn how to determine your threshold activity level and what steps you can take to reach it.

CONSTANT DIETING

We have become a nation of dieters. At any given time 40 percent of adults are dieting. Not only are we perpetual dieters but we are serial dieters as well. Surveys show the majority of dieters have been on two or more diets within the past 24 months. Yet, judged by any objective standards, our efforts to lose weight are a monumental failure. Depending on the survey, only 5 to 20 percent of people who lose more than 10 percent of their body weight keep it off for more than two years.

The one area that has been neglected in this discussion as to why diets fail is our genetic makeup. We do not have a weight-loss gene. To the contrary, all the mechanisms with regard to appetite and energy are specifically and efficiently designed to help us maintain our weight.

Consider again our Paleolithic ancestors. Food supply was erratic. Therefore, when food was available, there had to be a highly efficient mechanism to store it. The mechanisms that permit us to store excess food as fat are highly developed. Similarly, the mechanisms that encourage us to eat are far more developed than the mechanisms that tell us to stop eating. A large part of our central nervous system and gastrointestinal tract is specifically devoted to encouraging us to eat. Fast-forward a million years and you see how illogical it is to switch your body into a weight-losing, appetite-suppression mode.

Yo-Yo Dieting

It is well recognized that dieters lose and regain weight many times. Polls indicate that 31 percent of American women, ages 18 to 39, diet at least once a month. Yo-yo dieting results in cycles of weight loss from calorie restriction followed by weight gain. To determine the impact of yo-yo dieting on the body's metabolic adaptations, researchers simulated a yo-yo dieting pattern in animals.

As shown in Figure 4.4, in the first cycle of food restriction (left), the animals lost weight rapidly, and then when they resumed their normal patterns, they regained the weight. In the second cycle of food restriction (right), it took the animals twice as much time to lose the same amount of weight as in the first cycle, yet they regained the weight three times faster. In other words, during the second diet cycle, the energy circuit became far more efficient in converting food into additional weight. This study certainly explains the real-life experience of yo-yo dieters. But the issue goes beyond the matter of weight gain. The weight that is regained comes back mostly as fat. And the problem worsens as the percentage of body fat increases with each subsequent cycle.

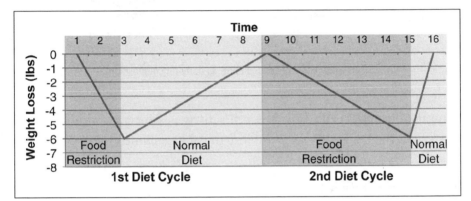

Figure 4.4. Effect of yo-yo dieting on weight loss and weight regain.

The impact of serial dieting on body fat composition was demonstrated in a study conducted by researchers at Arizona State University who compared body fat composition in two normal weight groups of women—one group had never dieted and the second group had on average dieted seven times in the previous 24 months. As shown in Figure 4.5 on the following page, although both groups were normal weight as measured by BMI, the serial dieters had 26 percent more body fat.

What these studies demonstrate is that when people lose and regain weight multiple times, negative changes occur in their body composition. Even if they manage to keep their weight under control through multiple rounds of dieting, they have a higher percentage of body fat than people of a similar weight who do not diet.

Yo-yo dieting has also been implicated in compromising the immune system. One study found that women who underwent more than five bouts of dieting had a much lower level of a specific type of immune cell called

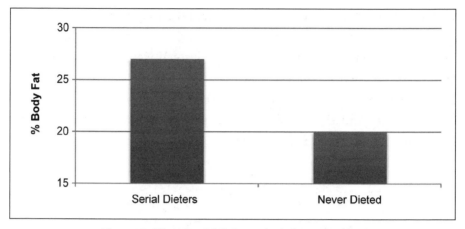

Figure 4.5. Effect of serial dieting on body-fat composition.

natural killer (NK) cells. Low NK cell activity is associated with increased cancer rates and a higher susceptibility to colds and infections.

The Caloric Deficit Paradox

An often-heard solution to the problem of obesity is to "eat less and move more." It sounds so simple and easy to do. Most of the commercial solutions and the recommendations of professionals, however, focus on the "eat less" part of the equation. To determine how much less one should eat, people turn to the Internet. Many websites have these nifty calculators. All you have to do is enter your current weight, your goal weight, and the number of calories you plan to reduce your diet by each day, and presto, it calculates how long it will take you to reach your goal weight.

Table 4.1 illustrates various recommendations of commercial programs, as well as a respected medical institution, the Mayo Clinic.

Since the average food consumption per day is 2,500 calories for women and 3,000 calories for men, following any of the total daily caloric recommendations above will produce a significant caloric deficit. Figure 4.6 illustrates the caloric deficit for men and women for the four popular plans noted in Table 4.1. All of them produce a caloric deficit greater than 1,000 calories. This sizable caloric deficit has little to do with how the fitness circuitry works but a lot to do with consumer expectations. Society

Table 4.1. Calorie Recommendations by Program

Plan	Daily Calorie Recommendation	
	Female	Male
Medifast	1,000	1,000
Mayo Clinic Plan	1,200	1,400
NutriSystem	1,200	1,500
Jenny Craig	1,300	1,300

demands instant gratification and weight loss is no exception. The greater the caloric deficit, the faster the pounds come off, or at least that would be the logical assumption. At a daily caloric deficit of 1,200 calories, a person loses a pound every three days. In order to lose ten pounds for that upcoming event, one simply has to start the diet 30 days beforehand.

The need for rapid weight loss has been perpetuated by obesity experts who suggest that people must lose five to seven pounds in the first two weeks of a diet, otherwise, they lose motivation and will go off the diet.

Nothing could be further from the truth. A caloric deficit of 500 or more calories per day almost guarantees diet failure. The greater the

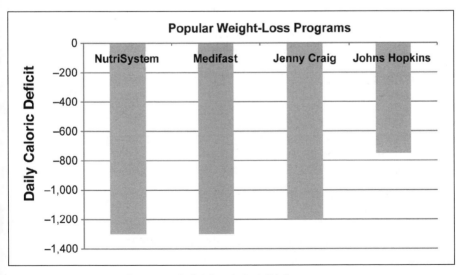

Figure 4.6. Ideal daily caloric deficit by program.

caloric deficit, the more difficult for long-term compliance and the faster the return to one's starting weight.

In the past five years, there has been resurgence in the use of very low calorie diets (VLCD). Although these diets should be used under a doctor's supervision, they often are not. A VLCD consists of prepackaged meals that total either 800 or 1,200 calories a day. This produces a very significant caloric deficit and, as you would expect, considerable short-term weight loss. What is interesting, however, is that studies comparing a VLCD that generated a caloric deficit of 1,800 calories per day to a more moderate caloric reduction diet of 750 calories per day produced almost the same dismal results over a year and a half (see Figure 4.7). Individuals on the VLCD lost more weight more quickly, but gained it back more quickly. The pattern of rapid weight loss and rapid weight gain represents the experience of almost every person who has gone on a diet. If one looks at how the fitness circuitry works in the context of the necessary adaptations critical for survival, it is easy to understand why.

It was essential that our Paleolithic ancestors maintain their body weight, particularly when food was in short supply. There had to be a balance among the energy necessary to stay alive, the resting energy expenditure, and the implications of breaking down muscle protein to meet energy needs. If Paleolithic man, when faced with long periods of food shortage,

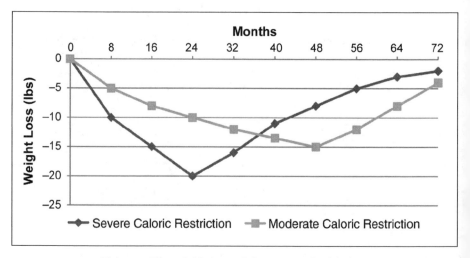

Figure 4.7. Effect of calorie restriction on rate of weight loss.

had to metabolize muscle for the necessary energy to maintain life, he would have compromised his ability to move, hunt, and ultimately survive.

To minimize the impact of a food shortage, an important adaptation exists in our hardwiring that was essential for our Paleolithic ancestor but which causes untold aggravation for individuals trying to lose weight. During a prolonged shortage of food or fasting, our resting metabolic rate drops. Scientists call this adaptive thermogenesis. This survival mechanism can be likened to a dimmer switch. If energy is in short supply, by dimming the lights, we can keep them on longer.

How Our Bodies Rebel Against Dieting

Adaptive thermogenesis is an integral part of the body's hardwiring and explains many of the frustrations of dieters. Dieters after two to three weeks find they stop shedding pounds even though they are faithfully adhering to their diet. In 1995, researchers from Rockefeller University published a study that explained the plateau effect. They showed that the resting energy expenditure in individuals on a diet could drop by 15 percent, or an equivalent of 250 to 300 calories per day. It is almost as if the body is playing a cruel joke on dieters. In their effort to lose weight quickly, dieters decrease their food intake to a level that is unsustainable long-term, and after two to three weeks, the body says, "Eat even less." The three-week weight-loss plateau is supported by other studies showing that the maximum decline in resting energy expenditure occurs at this time. No wonder dieters get discouraged!

As you have learned, the most fundamental property of the fitness circuitry is the high degree of integration among the circuits. In the presence of what the body perceives as a significant caloric deficit, the stress circuit is activated and cortisol is released.

Cortisol stimulates the breakdown of fat into energy, which is a good thing when we are trying to lose weight. However, other actions of cortisol have a profound negative effect on weight loss and overall fitness. If the calorie restriction is severe such as that seen with very low calorie diets, cortisol stimulates the breakdown of lean body mass while simultaneously strongly stimulating hunger sensations making it virtually impossible to stay on the diet. The combined effects of adaptive thermogenesis and acti-vation of the stress circuit is a lowering of the body's metabolism so you burn fewer calories at the same time you are hungrier. What does all this mean? That our bodies simply *do not like dieting.*

Rebound Weight Gain

It is frustrating enough for people who lose weight to simply regain the weight they lost, but most people actually gain back even more. Since diet-ing interferes with normal functioning of the circuitry, this dysfunction can continue long after the diet has ended. We have seen how adaptive thermo-genesis can limit weight loss, but it can also cause an increase in weight beyond the weight at which one started.

A typical scenario is a person substantially reduces caloric intake to lose weight. When the diet ends, he or she increases her food intake to a main-tenance level; unfortunately, the body hasn't gotten the memo. The effect of adaptive thermogenesis or reduction in resting energy expenditure can continue for 4 to 12 months after stopping the diet. In other words, even when eating in a maintenance mode, dieters are consuming more calories than their bodies are burning, which translates into weight gain that could exceed their previous weight.

The impact of this metabolic adaptation following significant weight loss is often either underestimated or ignored. Researchers at Rockefeller University studied daily energy requirements in 26 severely obese men and women following dieting in which the participants lost, on average, 114 pounds. After the weight loss, they found that the daily energy require-ments of the subjects were 25 percent lower than would have been antici-pated based on their post-dieting weight. Expressed another way, following a major drop in weight through dieting, a person would have to reduce his or her food intake 25 percent lower than a person of the same weight who had not dieted.

The Greater the Caloric Deficit, the Greater the Muscle Loss

An observation made almost 30 years ago is that people who lose a signifi-

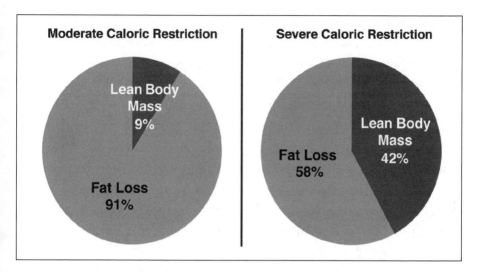

Figure 4.8. Effect of calorie restriction on fat and lean body mass loss.

cant amount of weight also lose significant amounts of lean body mass as well as fat.

Investigators at Rockefeller University looked at the impact of an increasing caloric deficit on body composition. The highest caloric deficit produced the greatest weight loss, as would be expected. What wasn't expected, however, was that the amount of fat loss remained constant and the amount of lean body mass loss increased in proportion to the caloric deficit. In other words, the higher the caloric deficit, the greater the loss in lean body mass. Just how dramatic these results are can be seen in Figure 4.8. At moderate calorie restriction (left), loss of lean body mass represented only 9 percent of the total weight loss. At severe calorie restriction loss (right), lean body mass represented 42 percent of the total weight lost. The loss of lean body mass reduces the level of fitness but also lowers the resting energy expenditure. A muscle cell burns seven times more energy than a fat cell. As lean body mass decreases, there is a concomitant decrease in resting energy expenditure, making it even more difficult to lose weight.

In the context of how the fitness circuitry works, it is not difficult to understand why weight is lost as muscle but comes back as fat. Following a period of calorie restriction, the circuitry hyper-adapts. Once normal food consumption is resumed, a dieter's body begins to increase fat storage, anticipating that another period of calorie restriction will occur.

Ironically, moderate to severe calorie restriction, which results in counter adaptations by the body, is unnecessary. This was shown in a recent study that compared the impact of low or moderate calorie restriction on weight loss. One group consumed a diet that had a daily caloric deficit of 200 calories. The second group had a daily caloric deficit of 750, which is generally the accepted recommendation. There was no difference in weight loss at six months between the two groups, in spite of the fact that one group was consuming 550 fewer calories per day. The investigators concluded that *lower reductions in energy intake may be as effective in achieving long-term weight loss as higher levels of restriction.*

This study shows that a small daily caloric restriction does not activate those countermeasures that limit weight loss, produce rapid weight regain, and increase the percentage of body fat.

Why Diet Drugs and Supplements Don't Work

When we diet, the fitness circuitry tries to rebalance our metabolism and, in doing so, makes it very difficult for a diet to succeed. When one tries to interfere with even a single circuit via drugs or supplements, a similar pattern emerges.

A major segment of the weight-loss market is supplements that reduce appetite. Although most of these supplements simply don't work, the ones that do work are capable of causing a transient disconnect or overload in the fitness circuitry. With time, the body will respond to the abnormal condition of not eating and the appetite circuit will be stimulated, thereby negating the effect of the supplement. Ephedra (ma huang), which at one time was one of the most popular weight-loss supplements, is an excellent example of how the body responds to appetite suppression. Even though ephedra became one of the most widely used supplements, there was never a single study published showing it had long-term effectiveness in reducing weight. Ultimately, ephedra was removed from the market because it was associated with a number of harmful side effects.

In 1992, a new prescription diet product was introduced that combined two constituents, phentermine and fenfluramine (popularly called fen-phen). It seemed like the ideal combination. Phentermine had been shown to decrease appetite while fenfluramine had been shown to increase satiety. In one combination, people had a drug that would reduce their appetite and when they ate would extend their feeling of fullness.

It was promoted as a miracle weight-loss product and soon became the number one prescription medicine in the United States, with sales in excess of $300 million. In 1997, it was withdrawn from the market because it was shown to cause heart valve disease. However, even prior to its removal, there was clear evidence from clinical studies that the body's mechanisms to prevent weight loss were activated. Studies showed that patients treated with phentermine and fenfluramine had a rapid decline in BMI over the first four months of treatment, after which the rate of decline slowed and then plateaued. There was little further weight loss after six months.

One of the most popular diet products available today is orlistat, which is available in both prescription (Xenical) and nonprescription (Alli) form. Orlistat works by preventing the absorption of fat. Taken with meals, orlistat increases the excretion of fat. This action causes a number of undesirable effects, but that is not the point here. Researchers noted that after a year, there was a plateau in weight loss in people taking orlistat. There was still a higher excretion of fat; therefore, the scientists knew the product was continuing to work.

Orlistat is a classic example of unintended consequences. Fat, particularly fat composed of long-chain fatty acids, plays a role in stimulating the body's major feel-full protein, CCK, a master switch (discussed earlier) that reduces hunger. By its action, both in the stomach and in the brain, CCK tells us to stop eating.

Researchers theorized that orlistat, by blocking the absorption of fat, was preventing the release of CCK and that is exactly what they found. CCK levels are decreased in individuals taking orlistat. Without the normal control of CCK on appetite, individuals taking orlistat over time began eating more thereby compensating for the fat calories that were lost through the action of orlistat.

Constant dieting has become a way of life. Yet, every time you diet, potent metabolic forces are activated within your body to almost guarantee that your diet will fail. The primary reason that dieting fails is not because of a lack of willpower or commitment but because dieting interferes with the body's natural metabolic rhythm. When you diet, your body activates a series of anti-diet measures, ranging from increased appetite to a loss of lean body mass to a reduction in your resting energy expenditure.

UNRESOLVED STRESS

Stress is part of the body's normal physiological rhythm. It plays an important role in providing a continual source of energy to the muscles as well as the short-term burst of energy required to respond quickly to a situation.

Cortisol, the stress hormone, rises during sleep, reaches a peak in the morning, and is generally low during the course of the day. However, our contemporary lifestyle has produced a marked change in the normal physiologic pattern of cortisol. We live in stressful times.

The increased stress manifests itself in higher levels of anxiety, but it also has a major impact on the normal functioning of our fitness circuitry. For example, consistently elevated levels of cortisol profoundly disrupt the energy circuit's ability to balance energy intake and energy expenditure; they also stimulate the hunger center of the brain to increase appetite while simultaneously stimulating the synthesis of fat, particularly in the abdominal region. Chronic stress is being increasingly recognized as a major factor in weight gain.

A sustained elevation in cortisol levels causes insulin resistance, the condition that characterizes type 2 diabetes. In the presence of insulin resistance, the body loses its ability to manufacture protein, resulting in a loss of lean body mass. Because of the effect of sustained levels of cortisol on lean body mass, appetite, and fat tissue, it is easy to understand why chronic stress has such a dramatic effect on the fitness circuitry. In Part Two, you will learn about steps you can take to minimize physiological and emotional stress.

NUTRITION CHOICES THAT IGNORE FUNCTION

Although what we eat is not the only determinant of how fit we are, it certainly plays a critical role. Unfortunately, diet dominates the fitness dialogue. Much of the debate has focused on only one aspect of fitness: weight, and the consequence has been to identify a magical ratio of macronutrients that will enable us to lose weight and become more fit. The various dietary recommendations by the American Heart Association (AHA), U.S. Department of Agriculture (USDA), American Diabetes Association, and others represent a confusing landscape—high fat/high protein, low fat/high carb, high protein/low carb, and so on.

A common theme in all the popular diets is to demonize a particular nutrient and make it the culprit for obesity. The first macronutrient to be singled out was fat; then it was carbohydrate. As might be expected, once a macronutrient is demonized, diets are introduced based on this publicity; thus, we have seen the popularity of low-fat diets wane, giving rise to low-carb diets. Figure 4.9 shows the recommended macronutrient composition of many popular diets.

The problem is that all these popular diet recommendations have the same fundamental flaw: they recommend a fixed macronutrient composition and this is simply *not how the body works*.

There is a functional rhythm in how the body uses macronutrients. There is an excellent rationale for the macronutrient composition recommended by the Ornish diet when energy needs are great or the Atkins diet

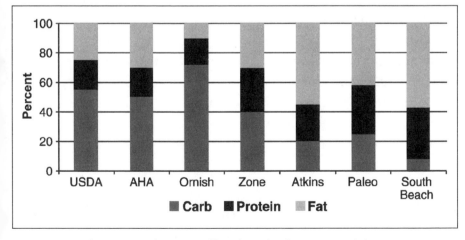

Figure 4.9. Nutrient composition of popular diet recommendations.

when the protein turnover circuit is active. But this just proves that even a broken clock will tell the correct time twice a day. These diets fail because they impose a rigid nutritional formula on an engine that requires a variable nutritional formula to operate at peak efficiency.

The impact of a fixed macronutrient composition on our fitness circuitry is significant. For example, a very low-carbohydrate intake will send a signal to the body to release cortisol. Although cortisol has beneficial effects, it can also cause an increase in appetite. High-fat diets can cause us to feel lethargic, potentially lowering our activity level below the appetite control threshold. High-protein diets can result in a higher percentage of protein being used for energy when fat and carbohydrate are far better sources.

By not synchronizing the composition of our meals to the body's natural metabolic rhythm, it becomes very difficult, if not impossible, to achieve our goal of fitness. A major study published in the *New England Journal of Medicine* compared all the popular diets. The results showed that there was no difference in weight loss over one year, and that the weight was modest in all cases—about four pounds.

Perhaps the best indicator of success is the National Weight Loss Registry, which tracks individuals who have lost more than 15 percent of their body weight and kept it off for two years or longer. In spite of the enormous popularity of the Atkins diet, there are only a handful of people on the National Weight Loss Registry who went on the Atkins diet and successfully kept the weight off.

The faulty thinking that underlies all popular diets is that what you eat is the sole determinant of your fitness and weight. Food is not the driver rather it is the integrated, efficient workings of your fitness circuits. The first focus should be on the engine—what makes it work and what makes it efficient. The second focus should be on fuel. If the carburetor in your car is faulty, changing your service station from Shell to Exxon will not make your car run better.

CHANGE IN SLEEP PATTERNS

We live in a 24/7 world. We shop 24/7. We buy food 24/7. We are entertained 24/7. This constant stimulation combined with longer commutes and extended working hours has significantly interfered with our normal sleep patterns. Over the last 50 years, the number of hours Americans are sleeping has declined from eight and half hours to seven hours a night. Numerous studies have shown that, as a consequence of this reduced sleep time, people are more tired, they have less energy, and they are less alert. That's to be expected. However, when we view these altered sleep patterns in the context of the body's biological clock, or circadian rhythm, the implications go far beyond just being tired. This biological clock is the master controller of your fitness level, and ultimately your overall health and longevity, so when you interfere with its normal rhythm, it has dramatic effects on the function of your fitness circuits.

The first evidence that changes in people's sleep patterns could dramatically alter their fitness circuitry came from a retrospective study that looked at the decline in sleep time since 1975 (Figure 4.10). Researchers noted that the curve representing the decrease in hours spent sleeping was almost a mirror image of the curve representing the increase in obesity. Researchers have now identified the mechanisms by which sleep deprivation disrupts the normal functioning of our circuitry.

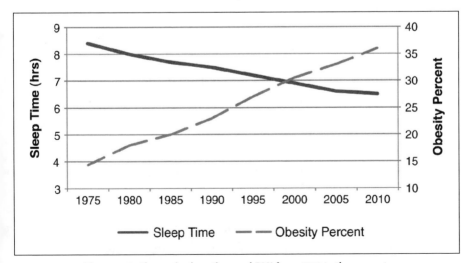

Figure 4.10. Change in sleep time and BMI from 1975 to the present.

Lack of Sleep Interferes with the Energy Circuit

Sleep plays an important role in maintaining normal function of the energy circuit, which explains why nighttime shift workers have an increased incidence of type 2 diabetes. Researchers have shown that when healthy subjects had less than four hours of sleep for six consecutive nights, their ability to metabolize glucose (sugar) was impaired and they had a higher level of insulin. In other words, sleep deprivation created the same physiological conditions as type 2 diabetes. Physiologically, this would translate into having less energy and an increased conversion of carbohydrate into fat. The impact of sleep deprivation on glucose metabolism was sustained throughout the next day.

Lack of Sleep Interferes with the Appetite Circuit

The association between sleep deprivation and increased BMI is very strong. In one study, 74 percent of the subjects who had an increase in their BMI also reported getting fewer than eight hours of sleep a night. Two well-designed studies shed light on this association. In one study subjects were either deprived of four hours' sleep or permitted to sleep for ten hours. Investigators measured the levels of two important appetite peptides: ghrelin (which makes you feel hungry) and leptin (which makes you feel full). They found that when subjects were sleep deprived, ghrelin increased 28 percent and leptin decreased 18 percent. The relationship between sleep and hunger was further confirmed in a 2009 study. Over a two-week interval, researchers measured daily levels of hunger in subjects who either received a normal night's sleep or were sleep deprived. The sleep-deprived subjects demonstrated a significant increase in daily hunger.

Lack of Sleep Interferes with the Stress Circuit

As you can imagine, sleep deprivation places physiologic stress on the body. Therefore, one would expect to see an impact on cortisol levels. This is exactly what researchers found. Following sleep deprivation, subjects sustained increases in cortisol levels that lasted two days.

Lack of Sleep Interferes with the Protein Turnover Circuit

When there is a daily caloric deficit greater than 500 calories, there is a disproportionate loss in lean body mass. In fact, the greater the caloric restriction, the greater the loss of lean body mass. Investigators from the University of Chicago examined the impact of sleep deprivation in two groups of subjects on a reduced-calorie diet. As shown in Figure 4.11, both groups lost similar amounts of weight (about 6.5 pounds), but the group who received five and a half hours of sleep a night lost 50 percent less fat than the group who had eight and a half hours of sleep.

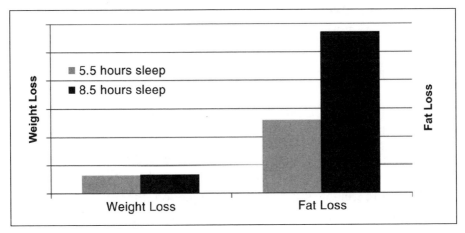

Figure 4.11. Effect of sleep deprivation on fat loss.

Get Fit, Sleep More?

It would be great if you could sleep your way to fitness. Unfortunately, that is not the conclusion of all these studies. Lack of sleep does, however, interfere with the natural rhythm of the fitness circuitry, and its impact is substantial. It is the only factor that disrupts the natural functioning of all four fitness circuits.

THE PERPETUAL MEAL

An enduring myth in weight loss is that consuming smaller meals more frequently during the day produces greater weight loss than consuming the same amount of calories in three meals. It sounds logical. Smaller meals would prevent a large spike in insulin, which is good, and smaller meals consumed more frequently would keep you more satisfied (if you are less hungry, you will eat less food). So, the theory goes. But the problem with this recommendation is that it's not supported by studies analyzing meal frequency patterns and caloric intake. In 1978, the average number of meals consumed per day was about 3.8. By 1996, it was almost 4.4. Interestingly, these surveys also showed that there was little change over the course of 20 years in the amount of calories people consumed at breakfast, lunch, and dinner. There was, however, a large increase in the number of calories people consumed as snacks. Calories consumed by snacking almost doubled to 423 calories per day.

More Meals, More Calories, More Weight

The small but frequent meal dogma is wrong, and following it may make it even more difficult to lose weight and get in shape. This recommendation is largely based on a single study in which overweight people consumed their daily calories in one meal or five meals. People on the five-meal regimen lost more weight. But on closer examination, the study protocol was badly flawed. More than ten subsequent studies have refuted the small but frequent meal hypothesis.

From an evolutionary perspective, the hypothesis makes no sense. Why would the body's circuitry operate more efficiently in the presence of more frequent eating times, when that is a condition that has only been satisfied in the United States and other developed countries in the last 50 years?

The small but frequent hypothesis was promulgated at almost the same time that the popular media began to demonize the hormone insulin. Its proponents claimed that smaller meals prevent an insulin peak. That is partially true. Yes, insulin levels peak after eating (the peak is related to the size of the carbohydrate content of the meal). However, insulin levels fall quite rapidly to normal levels in two to three hours. This represents an important physiological adaptation. On the other hand, a small elevation in insulin levels, which is seen following a small meal, profoundly inhibits the breakdown of fat.

Eating smaller meals, more frequently, also causes a sustained elevation of insulin over an extended period of time, which disrupts the body's ability to mobilize fat and use it for energy. Rather than increasing fat utilization, small and frequent meals actually increase the body's reliance on carbohydrate as a fuel source and block its use of fat.

The last argument against the small but frequent meal hypothesis has nothing to do with your circuitry but has much to do with your ability to accurately gauge the portion size of our meals. Studies have consistently shown that people underestimate the quantity of food that they eat. It's hard enough to accurately gauge portion sizes for three meals a day. It becomes that much harder when you are trying to gauge portion sizes for five or six meals a day. A small miscalculation can have a significant impact on weight gain. If an individual undercalculates by 20 calories per day, over a 20-year period, this will produce a weight gain of 40 pounds. It doesn't take much to throw the circuitry off. That 20-calorie miscalculation could move a normal weight (BMI 23.1) person into the overweight category (BMI 28.5).

WHY DIETS ALWAYS FAIL

Through diets, misguided nutritional advice, bogus products, and an unrealistic focus on weight loss rather than fitness, we have managed to interfere with the proper functioning of our fitness circuitry. When we overload a circuit, such as the appetite or energy circuit, and when we ignore the fact that the circuitry attempts to self-correct when it is damaged, we achieve a result that we don't want. There is a degree of arrogance that prevails in the popular and professional media that people can alter the way their fitness circuitry works without physiological consequences.

But the truth is, the mechanisms that maintain normal functioning of the fitness circuitry are incredibly strong and highly resistant to permanent change. This resistance to change, and the innate property of the fitness circuitry to rebalance itself, explains why diets fail. In the small percentage of cases where diets are successful, it is more a testament to individual willpower than to an artificial reprogramming of the circuitry. When faced with a reduced consumption of food, all four fitness circuits respond in a coordinated way that ultimately results in diet failure.

Table 4.2 summarizes the individual responses of the four circuits and the effect of these responses on our ability to lose weight. The more stringent the diet is in terms of calorie restriction, the greater the compensation by the individual circuits. These compensations are programmed into our DNA. Thus, the desire to eat increases, the deposition of fat increases, the body's resting metabolic rate (short- and long-term) declines, the conversion of food into fat increases, and lean body mass declines.

Table 4.2. Why Diets Always Fail— Response of the Fitness Circuits

Circuit	Response		Effect	
Stress	Cortisol	↑	Abdominal fat	↑
Appetite	Hunger peptides	↑	Desire to eat	↑
Energy	Energy utilization	↓	Short-term—resting metabolic rate	↓
	Energy storage	↑	Long-term—resting metabolic rate	↓
			% of food converted into fat	↑
Protein Turnover	Protein degradation	↑	Lean body mass	↓

When people diet, they are attempting to overcome the adaptations that are genetically programmed in their DNA. In the introduction, we likened this to pushing a large boulder uphill. Only a few people reach the fitness summit. The more likely scenario is that the large boulder rolls back downhill.

Don't let this information discourage you, however. Once you understand how your fitness circuitry works, this scenario can change dramatically. Because the adaptations for fitness are programmed into your genes, by simply providing the right conditions to allow your circuitry to work as designed, you can achieve your fitness goals. In other words, you are now rolling the boulder downhill. Chapter 5 will show you how easy it is to resynchronize and reconnect your fitness circuits.

Holiday Disconnection

Government surveys have shown that between the ages of 25 and 50, the average American gains one pound per year. The logical question is whether this one-pound gain occurs throughout the whole year or if it has a seasonal specificity. Almost everyone, whether they are overweight or not, would claim that during the holiday season, on average, they gain three to five pounds. This is an often-quoted statistic. Every year, as health writers draft their annual holiday weight-gain story, they repeat this statistic. Unfortunately, there is no documentation that substantiates the validity of the three- to five-pound holiday weight gain. A study published in the *New England Journal of Medicine* showed that this number is inflated.

The researchers measured the weights of nearly 200 adults in three time frames: the pre-holiday period from September to mid-November, the holiday period from mid-November to mid-January, and the post-holiday period from mid-January to mid-March. They showed that there is a holiday weight gain, but it is less than one pound. What is intriguing is that this study suggests that the one-pound weight gain per year occurs during the holiday season.

The question is whether changes during this period cause a disconnection or an overload of our fitness circuitry. On one hand, there is little doubt that most people consume more food during the holidays, which would explain a one-pound weight gain. However, the researchers also looked at activity levels. A high percentage of participants in this study were less active during the holiday period, and it is not surprising that an equally high percentage were also hungrier during this time. This suggests that during the holiday period, we may not reach the threshold level of activity necessary to ensure the proper functioning of our fitness circuitry. If this should occur, one would also expect an increase in appetite, which was, indeed, proven in this study.

The holiday disconnection would explain the weight gain, which is then exacerbated by actions often taken in the post-holiday period. January is called the "resolution month." It is the number one month for people to start diets and join health clubs, as they try to lose any excess weight gained over the holidays. Most people enter into this "get fit and lose weight" mode with great enthusiasm. They cut their daily caloric intake and begin a regular exercise program. As we have seen, dieting has a major impact on normal functioning of your fitness circuitry. It is not surprising that by June, any weight loss is regained and then some.

SUMMARY

Over the last 50 years, major changes in people's lifestyle, eating habits, and nutrition choices have impacted the normal functioning of the body's fitness circuitry. The major changes include not meeting the mandatory activity threshold, constant dieting, unresolved stress, excluding essential macronutrients from the diet, changes in sleep patterns, and eating small meals frequently throughout the day (the perpetual meal). A permanent change in a single factor can have a serious negative effect. Being aware of these factors brings you one step closer to resetting your fitness circuits.

CHAPTER 5

Resynchronizing and Resetting the Circuits

This chapter will show you how to resynchronize and reset the fitness circuits so that your metabolic machinery operates at peak efficiency. The resynchronizing process is neither difficult nor complicated, nor does it require a dramatic change in lifestyle. What is required, however, is that you pay attention to the details, as described in this chapter.

At one time, automobiles were not so complicated. They didn't require a computer to perform a tune up. You could optimize engine performance by adjusting a screw in the carburetor to make sure the mixture of air and gas was optimized. Then you used a timing light to adjust the distributor so that the fuel entered the pistons at just the right time to ensure maximum combustion and energy efficiency.

Although your body is far more complicated, the four steps to resynchronize your metabolic engine are quite simple. You don't have to rebuild the engine. You don't have to take measures to alter the way it functions. You simply have to make sure that it runs at optimum efficiency.

The secret is to recognize that you are hardwired to be fit. By making subtle changes in your daily activities and in meal timing and meal composition, you can resynchronize your body. In doing so, you take the first major step in transforming your body from being overweight and out of shape to what is its normal condition—fit and lean.

The four resynchronizers are:

1. Meeting your threshold level of activity.

2. Meeting your threshold level of sleep.

3. Timing meals to your body's natural functional rhythm.

4. Matching composition of your meals to your body's functional needs.

MEETING YOUR THRESHOLD LEVEL OF ACTIVITY

Think of daily activity as the current that drives your fitness circuitry. When the current is too low, the circuitry becomes dysfunctional. Similar to the way professionals have made "obesity" and "fitness" synonyms, experts have made "activity" and "exercise" synonymous. They are not. There are two types of activity: exercise and lifestyle activity.

Exercise is the activity that people do voluntarily. It involves increasing energy expenditure, usually for a finite period during the day. Exercise is sexy. It lends itself to public service commercials and "get out and exercise" initiatives featuring top athletes and celebrities. It makes for high-impact media, but it has a lower impact on resynchronizing the body than lifestyle activity. This is not to say that regular exercise cannot provide significant health benefits, which are discussed in Chapter 9. But to suggest that people cannot be fit without exercise is misleading.

The overwhelming majority of the world's population does not participate in regular exercise, and is not overweight and out of shape. What most of the world's population has in common with our Paleolithic ancestors is that they expend low levels of energy for most of the day through physical labor. Until the 1950s, blue-collar jobs were the norm. There is ample evidence suggesting our lack of fitness is not a result of eating more, but rather moving less.

In England, obesity rates have doubled over the last 20 years yet daily caloric intake appears to have decreased. At the turn of the century, the average American consumed more calories than we do today yet had a lower BMI. The emphasis on exercise is the result of a misguided focus on the first law of thermodynamics. If your exercise burns more calories than you eat, you lose weight. As you will see, this is a difficult goal to attain and ever more difficult to maintain.

This is why the second law of thermodynamics rules. The goal is to increase the efficiency of your engine. When your metabolic engine is operating at peak efficiency, energy expenditure, appetite, protein turnover, and stress are in balance.

We cannot achieve this balance unless we reach a minimum level of activity each day. As you may recall from Chapter 4, the research of Jean Mayer showed that when daily activity falls below a minimum level, there is an uncoupling of the appetite and energy circuits. When you are below the threshold level you gain weight because you are not burning off the calories you eat, but also because you eat more. This activity does not have to come in the form of exercise. Lifestyle activity is more important than exercise in helping people meet their threshold level.

Activity Should Be NEAT

Lifestyle activity is defined as the activity that people perform as part of their daily routines. As you can imagine, it is highly individualized. Lifestyle activity can range from sitting to commuting to gardening to vacuuming. Paleolithic man did not exercise, but his lifestyle activity levels were very high. Scientists have created an acronym to describe this lifestyle activity: It's called NEAT, which stands for non-exercise activity thermogenesis. NEAT is the physical activity all of us perform throughout the day that has nothing to do with exercise as we know it.

NEAT is the energy we burn when we fidget, walk to pick up the newspaper, run after our children, head to the refrigerator for a snack, and even stand while having our morning coffee. Earlier we pointed out that one's total energy expenditure consists primarily of two components: (1) resting energy expenditure, or the amount of energy necessary to maintain the body in a resting state, and (2) lifestyle energy expenditure, or NEAT, the amount of energy burned through lifestyle activities. NEAT can increase your total energy expenditure by as little as 20 percent of your resting metabolic rate if you have a very sedentary lifestyle, to as much as 200 percent of our resting metabolic rate if, for example, you work in construction. Table 5.1 on the following page gives the caloric expenditure of different activities.

Lifestyle activity plays a more important role in increasing your daily energy expenditure than exercise, because even if you exercise 30 minutes every day, which most people find hard to do, this only represents 4 percent of your waking time (assuming that approximately eight hours is spent

Table 5.1. Caloric Expenditure of Various NEAT Activities for 160 lb Male

Non-Exercise Activity	Net Calories Expended/Hour	Non-Exercise Activity	Net Calories Expended/Hour
Gardening	515	Typing on a computer	110
Walking the dog	245	Sitting talking on phone	82
Cooking	184		

sleeping). Thirty minutes of light to moderate exercise can burn about 150 to 200 calories per day. A small increase in energy expenditure taking place over 16 hours can greatly exceed 150 to 200 calories.

The importance of NEAT was demonstrated in a study conducted by researchers from the Mayo Clinic. They investigated changes in fat storage and energy expenditure in sixteen subjects who consumed 1,000 extra calories per day. They made sure that all the subjects exercised at a very low level during the study period. They found a significant variation in the amount of weight gain among the subjects even though they were consuming the same amount of extra calories over their resting caloric needs. Although they controlled caloric expenditure and exercise activity, they did not control NEAT activity among the subjects. As you might expect, there is a wide range of NEAT activity. Some of us fidget, some of us pace, and some of us walk briskly, while others sit very still or stroll, just to name a few of the ways NEAT varies among individuals. The researchers found there was a strong negative correlation between the amount of NEAT and weight gain. In other words, people in the study who had a higher NEAT burned more of the extra calories, and the higher the NEAT, the less weight gain resulted from overeating.

These same investigators also used a highly sophisticated technique to measure energy expenditure by different NEAT activities. As shown in Figure 5.1, when compared with lying down, sitting increased energy expenditure by 4 percent, fidgeting while seated by 54 percent, standing motionless by 13 percent, and fidgeting while standing by 94 percent. Walking at one mile per hour increased energy expenditure by 154 percent.

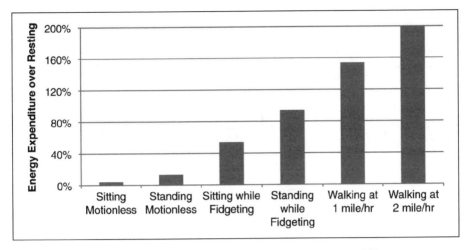

Figure 5.1 Energy-expenditure comparison of various NEAT activities.

The increase in energy expenditure shown by different NEAT activities was similar regardless of whether the subjects were normal weight or obese. In other words, increasing NEAT activities play an important role in helping you become fit.

Figure 5.2 on the following page shows the impact of a small increase in NEAT or lifestyle activity versus 30 minutes of exercise per day. A sedentary person who exercises can expect to see an increase in daily energy expenditure over an individual who doesn't (2,440 calories vs. 2,274 calories). However, even a small change in lifestyle activity, for example, increasing standing time per day, can result in a total daily caloric expenditure greater than that seen with just adding exercise (2,476 calories vs. 2,440 calories). Small changes in one's daily activity pattern can produce large increases in total energy expenditure. Although exercise offers additional benefits in terms of fitness (see Chapter 9), the example does show, however, that brief bouts of exercise may not be sufficient from a total energy perspective.

In 1999, investigators from Johns Hopkins University published a one-year study comparing the effect of lifestyle activity versus exercise in 40 obese women. All the subjects were on a low-fat diet of 1,200 calories per day. One group participated in aerobic classes three times a week that expended about 500 calories per workout. The second group was encouraged to increase their lifestyle physical activity by 30 minutes per day by

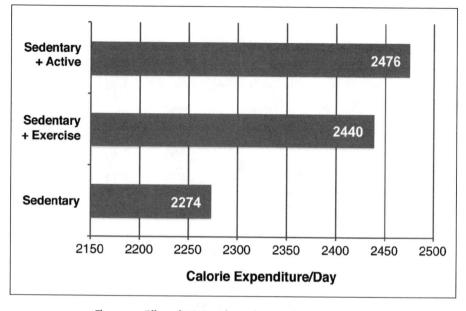

Figure 5.2. Effect of NEAT and exercise on caloric expenditure.

walking instead of driving and taking the stairs instead of the elevator. After 16 weeks, weight loss between the two groups did not differ significantly, and, interestingly, after one year the subjects who had increased their lifestyle activity maintained greater weight loss than the group who exercised.

In a more recent study, investigators analyzed the relationship between intensity of physical exercise and body fat in 81 women between the ages of 48 and 55. They used a device to measure the amount of time each subject spent in physical activities ranging from sedentary to vigorous. They noted there was no correlation between body fat and the amount of time spent in either moderate or vigorous activity. They did find that there was a strong relationship between the amount of time spent in light physical activity and the amount of body fat. Women who spent the most time performing moderate physical activity, or NEAT, had 20 percent lower body fat than women who were more sedentary. These studies do not suggest that there is not significant fitness benefits derived from exercise, but rather lifestyle activity plays an essential role in attaining the critical threshold level.

A growing body of science suggests that obesity results from an increase in a sedentary lifestyle. On average, overweight people sit 152 minutes more per day than normal weight people. Being sedentary is recognized as a separate health risk factor. For example, people with predominantly sedentary lifestyles who also exercise are at a greater risk for future health problems than people who have slightly more active lifestyles but do not exercise. NEAT represents an effective way to raise daily activity levels above the activity threshold level, thereby helping to resynchronize the fitness circuitry.

You Can't Bank Daily Lifestyle Activity

The body's master clock resets itself every 24 hours. Think of your daily lifestyle activity as the currents that keep this master clock running. Increased activity yesterday has no carryover effect today. Your circuitry can't function properly if the supply of current is erratic. That's why it's essential that you make the subtle changes in your lifestyle to insure that you reach your threshold level each and every day.

What Is Your Threshold Level?

Your threshold level of activity is a function of your age, weight, and height. For example, a 40-year-old, 140-pound woman who is 5 feet 7 inches tall would have a threshold level of activity of 695 calories per day. In other words, this individual would have to expend 695 calories per day in excess of her resting caloric expenditure. An expenditure of 695 calories through lifestyle activity is the minimum level of activity necessary for efficiency functioning of your fitness circuitry. In Chapter 9, you will learn a simple way to determine the threshold level that is ideal for you.

MEET YOUR THRESHOLD LEVEL OF SLEEP

Once you recognize the critical role circadian rhythm plays in controlling metabolic, physiological, and behavioral function, it becomes much easier to understand why sleep is an important factor in resynchronizing your circuitry. We are not nocturnal creatures. We are programmed to be active during the day. As we extend our day into the evening, we disrupt every one of the circuits necessary for determining our level of fitness. Sleep deprivation causes the appetite, energy, protein turnover, and stress circuits to become dysfunctional. There is a strong correlation between sleep deprivation and type 2 diabetes, obesity, and body composition to name just a few. Scientists have now identified the specific biologic mechanisms that are altered during periods of sleep deprivation. The key question is what should be your threshold level for sleep? When sleep time is reduced to five hours or less it alters all four of the fitness circuits. However, these changes do not take place when sleep time is seven and a half hours or more. Studies have also shown that the detrimental effects of sleep deprivation can be normalized within one week of normal sleep patterns.

The focus of this book is that through fitness you achieve a wide range of health benefits. This is particularly relevant with regard to meeting your threshold level of sleep. For example, scientists have noted that there is a relationship between certain cardiovascular incidents and time of death. Heart attacks and strokes tend to occur in early morning hours. There is good evidence to suggest that this is not merely coincidence. Sleep deprivation increases a metabolic marker of inflammation called C-reactive protein. Higher levels of C-reactive protein, which means higher levels of inflammation, have now been identified as a risk factor in cardiovascular disease. Higher levels of inflammation that are maintained over long periods of time have been suggested as a cause of obesity. Getting seven to seven and a half hours of sleep each night is an essential component in resetting and resynchronizing your circuitry.

TIME MEALS TO YOUR BODY'S NATURAL FUNCTIONAL RHYTHM

The master clock in our brain controls and coordinates the functioning for each of the four circuits. Each circuit has a unique rhythm that is based on achieving optimum metabolic efficiencies. For example, since the body is programmed to be active during daylight hours, the energy circuit operates at peak activity during the day when energy needs for locomotion and muscle activity are greatest.

On the other hand, creation of lean body mass is an energy-requiring process. If the protein circuit were activated during the day, it would be competing with the energy circuit. This is not particularly efficient, and by now, the one thing you can be most certain about is that your body is very efficient when it comes to energy conservation. As energy needs decline during the course of the day, the protein turnover circuit becomes more active. In other words, it is easier to build protein and lean body mass during the evening than it is during the day.

The importance of circadian rhythm to meal timing can best be illustrated by a 2009 study published in *Obesity*. The investigators compared the effects of feeding mice a high-fat diet in the evening versus in the daytime. Both groups were given the same number of calories over a 24-hour period and the investigators made certain that activity levels were equal in the two groups. What they found is that the mice, which are nocturnal creatures, gained 58 percent more weight when fed a high-fat diet during the daylight hours than mice fed the same diet during the night. The authors concluded that the synchrony "between circadian and metabolic processes plays an important role in the regulation of energy balance and body weight control." In other words, eating at the wrong time can lead to weight gain.

Similar results have been seen in human trials. In one study, researchers noted there was high correlation between obesity and a shifting of eating patterns to the evening hours. A 2008 study looked at nighttime eating and followed the subjects over five years. They found that nighttime eaters gained almost three times more weight than non-nighttime eaters. All these studies clearly show that *when* we eat can have a dramatic effect on overall metabolic efficiency.

MATCH THE COMPOSITION OF YOUR MEALS TO YOUR BODY'S FUNCTIONAL NEEDS

This resynchronizer was relatively unimportant to our Paleolithic ancestors. They ate what was available: it could be berries, it could be meat. Any loss of metabolic efficiency that resulted from the fact that meal composition was not synchronized to function was more than compensated for by their high level of daily activity.

For many of us, our activity level does not reach our threshold level. Therefore, marrying what we eat to the specific functional interval can have enormous impact on metabolic efficiencies. This approach is simply logical. During the functional interval when energy needs are the highest, it would make sense to consume meals that could be easily converted into usable energy.

There are four functional intervals during each 24-hour cycle. Each interval is characterized by a different primary function, which means the body's nutritional requirements change during the day in a predictable way. More will be said about our four functional intervals in the next chapter. We also know that each of the three macronutrients—carbohydrate, fat, and protein—have a primary metabolic function. Carbohydrates are used for rapid energy; fats, for sustained energy and appetite suppression; and proteins, for repairing and rebuilding lean body mass. It's logical that the greatest metabolic efficiency is achieved when what people eat is matched to the body's functional intervals.

You see an excellent example of this when you start up your car in the morning. The automobile engine uses a combination of air and fuel. When the engine is cold, it requires a higher percentage of fuel. As the car warms up, the engine burns a higher percentage of oxygen. In other words, it becomes a leaner mixture. On the highway, the fuel mixture becomes even leaner.

Your fitness engine works in a similar way. Each of the fitness circuits requires different combinations of macronutrients in order to function optimally. During the course of the day, different circuits are selectively turned on. To ensure that the fitness circuitry is always operating at peak efficiency, you must change the mixture of carbohydrate, protein, and fat. Failure to recognize this fact is the fundamental flaw in almost every popular diet today. In the next chapter, you will learn how your body changes functionally throughout a 24-hour period and what you can do to fuel it efficiently.

SUMMARY

Changes in our lifestyle, eating habits, and nutrition have created a dysfunctional fitness circuitry. Although the fitness circuits have a remarkable ability to respond to dramatic changes in the environment, we have exceeded the capacity of this remarkable machinery to resynchronize itself. Fortunately, resynchronization is not difficult. It involves the four key steps discussed in this chapter: (1) meeting your threshold level of activity, (2) meeting your threshold level of sleep, (3) timing your meals to your body's natural functional rhythm, and (4) matching the composition of your meals to your body's functional needs. Taking this action allows your fitness machinery to operate at peak efficiency. In Part Two, you will learn how to put this program into action.

CHAPTER 6

The Functional Day

We use different criteria to segment our 24-hour day. The criteria can be as simple as daytime and nighttime. More commonly we segment our day by activity—work, leisure, and sleep or eating times—breakfast, lunch, and dinner or both.

One of the more profound social changes occurring in the last 50 years has been the blurring together of what formerly were very distinct daily segments. Take meal times, for example. Five hundred years ago, people ate two meals per day: a light meal around sunup, and the main meal between noon and 2:00 P.M. In the 1500s, the affluent members of society added a third meal called supper, which was consumed between 8:00 P.M. and 10:00 P.M.

The three-meal segmentation worked well for the last 450 years. Interestingly, the three-meal segmentation is closely synchronized with the body's natural rhythm, particularly since people's daily lifestyle activity levels were higher and on average they slept more than eight hours each night. That's no longer the case. Food is always available and is more portable thanks to drive-in restaurants and the many snack food options. Eating times are often determined by an increasingly erratic and hectic schedule. The same holds true for our daily activities. In a 24/7 world where we can shop or work whenever we desire, daily activity has moved into the evening hours, often intruding on our sleep time. Additionally, we have seen a decline in lifestyle activity as we have become more sedentary.

The net result of these changes is that our activity, sleep, and eating patterns are out of sync with the body's natural physiological rhythm and, as we have seen, this has unintended and detrimental consequences on our level of fitness.

ACTIVITY, TIMING, AND NUTRITION

The research that we, along with other colleagues, conducted with elite athletes and seniors (discussed in the Preface) clearly demonstrated that three essential conditions were necessary to enable the fitness circuits to work in an ultra-efficient mode. They were timing, activity, and the right combination of nutrients. Once these three conditions were satisfied the circuitry operated in an ultra-efficient mode. To place this in perspective, in an ultra-efficient mode, protein synthesis, which is a prerequisite for building lean body mass, could increase almost threefold.

Each of the four circuits that determine your level of fitness has a unique and predictable 24-hour rhythm that is controlled by your body's master clock. As shown in Figure 6.1, at any given hour of the day, the body's net metabolic activity results from the composite activity of each of the four fitness circuits.

Circuitry integration assures that the four circuits act in a coordinated way avoiding a metabolic impasse that would result when the actions of one circuit negated the actions of another. For example, when the body's energy needs are highest, the protein turnover circuit operates at a low level. When one examines the patterns of each circuit over 24 hours, as illustrated in Figure 6.1, it is evident that our 24-hour day can be segmented into four functional intervals:

1. Restoration Interval: 7:00 A.M. to 9:00 A.M.

2. Activity Interval: 9:00 A.M. to 5:00 P.M.

3. Rebuilding Interval: 5:00 P.M. to 11:00 P.M.

4. Sleep Interval: 11:00 P.M. to 7:00 A.M.

Not only is each functional interval defined by a specific time segment of the day, but it is also defined by a principle metabolic activity. For example, from 11:00 P.M. to 7:00 A.M., the stress circuit is most active; from 9:00 A.M. to 5:00 P.M., the energy circuit is most active. Keep in mind

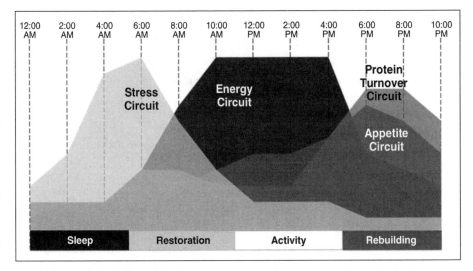

Figure 6.1. 24-hour rhythm of stress, energy, protein turnover, and appetite circuits.

that these intervals are not fixed in stone. There is individual variation in the timing of the four functional intervals. For example, you can eat breakfast between 6:00 A.M. and 9:30 A.M., and it will have the same beneficial effect. Once you are aware of the timing of each interval, synchronizing your daily activity and meals to these functional intervals gives you a valuable tool in your quest for fitness.

The next section describes each functional interval in terms of circuit activities and nutritional considerations.

RESTORATION INTERVAL

The Restoration Interval begins around daybreak. It follows the longest interval of the day that the body goes without food and without physical activity. Since the body has to maintain minimal function while asleep, it is forced to call upon energy reserves stored in muscle and fat cells. The master switch involved is cortisol. Just prior to daybreak, cortisol levels are at their highest of the day. Because energy stores are depleted during the night the hunger pathways is activated.

Every 24 hours the body's master clock is reset, which means that from an energy perspective the Restoration Interval is critical. This phase not only re-primes the metabolic machinery to enable you to start the day, but it also provides long-term effects that extend for the succeeding 12 to 15 hours. Of all the meals that you eat, nutrition consumed in the two hours after you awaken is the most satiating or satisfying meal of the day.

In a study conducted at the University of Texas at El Paso, investigators measured the relative satiating qualities of breakfast, lunch, and dinner. They found that breakfast was the most satiating meal of the day and dinner the least satiating. Other studies have confirmed the benefits of consuming food during the Restoration Interval on appetite regulation throughout the day. Researchers have found that people who eat breakfast consume fewer calories over the remainder of the day than people who skip breakfast. This translates into greater weight loss. Vanderbilt University researchers measured weight loss in two groups, each consuming the same amount of calories. One group consumed the calories in two meals, but skipped breakfast. The second group consumed the calories in three meals, including breakfast. After 12 weeks, the breakfast eaters lost almost 50 percent more weight than the no-breakfast group.

Other researchers have validated the importance of consuming nutrition during the Restoration Interval. A 1996 study examined whether food, eaten predominately in the morning, affected changes in body weight versus food consumed later in the day. Although total calories were equal in both groups, the group that ate their food predominately in the morning lost 16 percent more weight. These studies show that there is a strong correlation between long-term weight loss and eating during the Restoration Interval. It is interesting to note that 78 percent of successful dieters (those who lost more than 10 percent of their body weight and kept if off for two years) reported eating breakfast every day.

Eat a Bigger Breakfast—Lose More Weight

Perhaps the most compelling study on the critical role of the Restoration Interval was reported in 2008. The study was conducted over eight months and compared two groups of obese women. The first four months focused on weight loss and the second four months on weight maintenance. One group ate a low-carbohydrate diet that totaled 1,085 calories per day. For this group, breakfast was the smallest meal of the day. The second group consumed a high-carbohydrate diet that totaled 1,285 calories per day. For the high-carbohydrate, higher calorie group, breakfast was the largest meal of the day. Conventional thinking would suggest that the group eating more calories would lose less weight. Based on media infatuation with low-carbohydrate diets, one would have also expected the high-carbohydrate group to fare even worse. The results were dramatic and surprising: after eight months, the low-carbohydrate group lost 10 pounds; the high-carbo-hydrate, big-breakfast group lost 37 pounds.

Although it is not known precisely why eating during the Restoration Interval provides so many metabolic benefits, researchers have shown that food consumed during this interval raises a person's metabolic rate. When the body's metabolic rate is elevated, it results in a better balance between energy expenditure and energy consumption.

In spite of the well-documented benefits of eating during the Restoration Interval, studies indicate that 40 percent of the population skip breakfast regularly and as many as 60 percent skip breakfast at least one time during a month. The numbers for teenagers are even higher. It is not surprising that adolescent obesity is becoming a major health concern.

Optimizing Nutrition for the Restoration Interval

The body's metabolic status upon awakening is characterized by a depletion of energy stores and protein resulting from higher levels of cortisol. Carbohydrates are the ideal macronutrient to replenish muscle energy stores. Additionally, carbohydrate consumption reduces cortisol levels. These beneficial effects of carbohydrate are lost on people who skip breakfast. If high cortisol levels are maintained, the body continues to break down muscle protein through the mid-morning hours. The other macronutrient required during the Restoration Interval is protein, which is essential to replace the muscle protein that may have been broken down for energy while we were sleeping.

Consuming the right combination of nutrition during the Restoration Interval will enable you to have better appetite control throughout the day, while at the same time providing you with more energy for physical and mental activities.

ACTIVITY INTERVAL

We are programmed to be active during daylight hours, which are generally between 9:00 A.M. and 5:00 P.M. During this time interval, the energy
circuit reaches its maximum level of efficiency as long as one other essential criterion is met: we must be expending sufficient calories through
lifestyle activities to ensure that the body's energy expenditure is balanced
with its energy intake. This means that physical activity during the Activity Interval has the greatest impact on our path to fitness. Conversion of
carbohydrates to energy is far more efficient during the Activity Interval.
Almost 50 years ago, British researchers showed that carbohydrate utilization was most efficient at 9:00 A.M., and declined in the afternoon and
evening. Similar results have been noted in individuals who work at night.
Carbohydrates consumed at night are not as efficiently converted into
energy as carbohydrates consumed during the day. As might be expected,
nighttime workers have a much higher incidence of obesity and type 2 diabetes—one of the clinical consequences of obesity.

Efficient conversion of carbohydrates, however, does not take place if
you fail to reach your threshold level of activity. Recall Dr. Mayer's work.
When lifestyle activity is elevated, there is a tight balance between energy
consumption and energy expenditure. When you are sedentary, there is an
uncoupling between your appetite and your energy expenditure. In the
absence of a minimum amount of physical activity, you not only convert
more of your food to fat, but you also eat more because you are hungrier.

Optimizing Nutrition for the Activity Interval

During the Activity Interval, the fitness circuitry works in a coordinated
fashion to maximize energy production for muscle movement. Since carbohydrates are the ideal nutrient to provide muscle energy, carbohydrate consumption should be quite high during this interval. (Muscle energy
requirements during this interval represent from 70 to 90 percent of the
body's energy needs.) Similarly, protein consumption should be low. The
metabolic processes responsible for manufacture and repair of protein
require energy. Since muscle energy requirements have the highest priority
for the cell, the protein turnover circuit is relatively inactive during the day.

REBUILDING INTERVAL

The Rebuilding Interval between 5:00 P.M. and 11:00 P.M. represents the best time to stimulate protein synthesis. Since protein synthesis is an energy-requiring process, it makes little metabolic sense for it to take place between 9:00 A.M. and 5:00 P.M. when the fitness circuitry is working overtime to maximize energy production. As shown in Figure 6.1, as activity of the energy circuit falls in late afternoon, the protein turnover circuit activity rises. Additionally, people become hungrier in the evening. From a functional perspective, during the Rebuilding Interval, you want to maximize protein synthesis and minimize feelings of hunger.

Optimizing Nutrition for the Rebuilding Interval

Consuming a high-protein meal during the Rebuilding Interval provides multiple benefits. Even though the apparatus that builds protein during this interval is turned on, it still requires a source of raw materials in the form of ingested protein. Eating a high-protein meal during the rebuilding interval can double protein synthesis.

You can also get an additional protein-building benefit if you exercise in the late afternoon. You will see in Chapter 9 why, because of the body's circadian rhythm, late afternoon is the best time to exercise. If consuming your rebuilding meal takes place after your exercise, you can triple protein synthesis. Protein also decreases appetite, a particularly important consideration, since the evening hours from 5:00 P.M. to 8:00 P.M. are a prime time for consuming extra calories.

SLEEP INTERVAL

The interrelationship between sleep deprivation and fitness is well documented. Sleep loss is associated with increased hunger, sustained levels of stress, and obesity. The negative effects of sleep deprivation, especially on the conversion of food into energy, are seen quickly. Following four nights of just four hours sleep a night, researchers from the University of Chicago found that the subjects' response to a high-carbohydrate meal was similar to that observed in type 2 diabetics.

Exercise—The Fifth Functional Interval

Each of the four functional intervals is regulated by the body's internal circadian clock. Each interval activates different fitness circuits so that they function at optimal efficiency. Although exercise is not controlled by this clock—since we can exercise at any time of the day—it shares an important attribute of the four functional intervals. Like them, exercise increases the sensitivity of the fitness circuits. It increases the muscles' ability to respond to nutrition and increases protein turnover. Exercise improves appetite control and raises energy levels while reducing stress. Although the fitness circuits can be brought back into balance without a regular exercise program, improvements in body composition and overall fitness are going to occur more readily if you are willing to commit to three to four short exercise sessions a week. In Chapter 9, you'll learn more about the specific effects of exercise on the fitness circuits and overall health.

We cannot minimize the importance of the Sleep Interval in maintaining your overall health, as well as in helping you achieve your level of fitness. It appears that the proper amount of sleep needed varies from person to person, but studies suggest that a person's threshold level of sleep should be at least seven and a half hours per night. Our hectic and overscheduled lives often result in getting less than the threshold level. The result: we generate a sleep debt. Unfortunately, you can't pay off a sleep debt easily. Losing a total of five hours' sleep over a week can't be made up on the weekend by sleeping five hours more. This extra sleep only reduces the sleep debt by 20 to 30 percent.

Just as your threshold level of activity is essential for proper functioning of the fitness circuitry, so is your threshold level of sleep. The Sleep Interval also illustrates why stress, generated as a natural consequence of the circadian rhythm, is essential to your health and well-being by maintaining critical physiological functions. The body is conditioned to handle stress generated as part of the normal circadian cycle. Unfortunately, it is not as well equipped in dealing with the psychological and emotional stresses so prevalent in everyday life. Stress is a key desynchronizer of fitness circuitry. As touched on earlier, there is substantial research showing that chronic stress is a major causative factor of obesity. Although the body naturally regulates stress levels generated as a consequence of its circadian rhythm, we need to have additional mechanisms that help us control the stress of daily life. There is no single answer for everyone. The inset below describes some of the best methods to relieve stress. Find the ones that work for you and train yourself to recognize when stress levels are high so you can take the appropriate action.

The Best Ways to Relieve Stress

1. Take a long walk in a nature setting.

2. Take deep breaths.

3. Take a long hot shower.

4. Exercise.

5. Cook a meal.

6. Learn something new.

7. Get a pet.

8. Talk to someone.

9. Dance to your favorite music.

10. Ask for help with jobs you dislike.

11. Unclutter your surroundings.

12. Stand up and stretch.

13. Clean out your closet.

14. Get enough sleep.

15. Sing along with music.

16. Take a walk with a friend.

17. Strive for excellence, not perfection.

18. Do everything in moderation.

19. Stop saying negative things to yourself.

20. Look at problems as challenges.

21. Walk in the rain.

22. Avoid negative people.

23. Simplify meal times.

24. Set priorities in your life.

25. Anticipate your needs.

26. Draw a picture.

27. Take a mini vacation.

28. Learn to say no to demands on your time.

29. Take a nap.

30. Take a drive in your car.

Optimizing Nutrition for the Sleep Interval

You might be asking, "What possible nutritional considerations should I be concerned with while I'm sleeping?" There is considerable evidence showing that people who wake up and eat during the night have a much higher incidence of obesity. Therefore, nighttime eating is not a nutritional recommendation during the 24-hour day. However, drinking a high-protein beverage just prior to sleep can provide an important benefit by reducing the breakdown of muscle protein while you sleep.

SUMMARY

Although we may divide our day in terms of meal timing, activity, and light/dark cycles, the body's master clock, which is programmed into our DNA, segments every 24-hour period into four functional intervals. Each functional interval represents the composite activity of the four fitness circuits. The intervals and the specific times in which they are most active include:

1. Restoration Interval: 7:00 A.M. to 9:00 A.M.

2. Activity Interval: 9:00 A.M. to 5:00 P.M.

3. Rebuilding Interval: 5:00 P.M. to 11:00 P.M.

4. Sleep Interval: 11:00 P.M. to 7:00 A.M.

Because each of these intervals has a primary functional activity, synchronizing when you eat, what you eat, and when you are most active to these four functional intervals will optimize how efficiently they work.

CHAPTER 7

Resolutions for Success

L iving a lifestyle that promotes fitness is far more complicated today than it was for our Paleolithic ancestors. When fitness and survival are so intimately linked as they were for early man, there are not many personal choices. This, of course, is not the case today. We have so many choices, many of which create barriers to achieving the level of fitness that we desire. The faulty choices we make can more than cancel out our circuitry's ability to keep us fit.

The Hardwired Fitness Program is a powerful way to reprogram your body, but unfortunately, the circuitry does not necessarily reprogram your mind or your attitudes, which are equally important in determining whether you achieve your fitness goals. Additionally, the changes that you must make mentally are contrary to much of the media and commercial propaganda with which people are bombarded every day.

Before you begin the Hardwired Fitness Program in Part Two, there are five resolutions you should make. Unlike your New Year's resolutions, which are made on January 1 and usually broken by January 15, these are resolutions that you make for life.

Resolution #1 "I Will Never Diet Again"

In a nation so committed to dieting, this may be the hardest resolution to make. But, as detailed in this book, there is overwhelming science that proves that not only does dieting not work, but it also results in greater long-term weight gain. Dieting can produce significant short-term reductions equal to 10 to 20 percent of your starting weight. However, the process by which this weight is lost mobilizes multiple circuits in your body to compensate for this short-term weight loss. Your body's metabolic mechanisms to prevent weight loss are efficient and unrelenting. Dieting is like trying to hold your breath. You may be able to do it for a minute, but any interruption in oxygen ignites a series of metabolic responses in your body that force you to breathe. Whether through a meal plan, drug, or supplement, dieting is an artificial contrivance similar to holding your breath.

This resolution requires constant vigilance on your part. Weight-loss ads are seductive. The case studies that are featured are not reflective of reality. Think about all the high-profile celebrities who have endorsed the various diet products and programs over the years. Even with their cadre of trainers, nutritionists, and consultants supplied by the commercial sponsor, many of these high-profile celebrities regain the weight and quickly disappear from the ads. The next time they are seen is usually in a celebrity magazine, and they have regained the weight and then some.

So when you think, "This time will be different," you might wish to refer back to Table 4.3 on page 57, which shows the many different ways the body will fight your dieting efforts.

Resolution #2   "I Will Be Patient"

When you live in a society that thrives on instant gratification, it is not surprising that the promise of losing 10 pounds in a week is very attractive. To achieve that promise, people who are overweight are willing to endure almost anything and to spend what it takes. Although accurate figures on how much the United States spends on dieting solutions is difficult to come by, it is estimated that sales of products specifically focused on weight loss approach $100 billion per year. This includes foods, low-calorie beverages, weight-loss plans, supplements, and the like. It has also been estimated that at any given time almost 120 million Americans are on a diet. This works to a per capita expenditure of over $800 per year per person.

Fundamental to almost every diet product, plan, or book is instant weight loss. For most, it took years to gain the weight. The Hardwired Fitness Program will not guarantee you instant success. We cannot guarantee three-, four-, or five-week success, but we can guarantee that if you follow the principles outlined in this book, you will see dramatic changes in your fitness level in 24 weeks. And, most important, these changes can be permanent because you are resynchronizing the circuits that control whether or not you are fit.

Resolution #3   "I Will Take Advantage of Every Opportunity to Increase My Daily Lifestyle Activity"

The importance of non-exercise activity, or lifestyle activity, must not be underestimated. The adaptation that exists within our DNA is for low-intensity activity for sustained periods. A recent study published in the *Journal of the American College of Sports Medicine* showed that low-level lifestyle activity may provide greater caloric, health, and longevity benefits than exercising for 30 minutes per day, three or four times a week, even if the physical activity exceeds daily recommendations. This study verifies the work conducted more than 50 years ago, demonstrating that a minimum level of activity is critical for the proper functioning of the fitness circuitry.

When you create a Personal Energy Inventory as outlined in Chapter 8, don't be surprised if you have a preponderance of net-zero activities— in other words, activities that provide no incremental energy benefit over your resting energy expenditure. These are opportunities, not chores. For example, stand up while you are working. At lunchtime walk to your favorite restaurant. When you watch television, do some stretching. You can think up and perform creative ways to increase your lifestyle activity and achieve your threshold level. With a little imagination, you will find it easy to incorporate additional lifestyle activity into your daily life, and you might even find it enjoyable.

Resolution #4 "I Will Add Functionality to My Meal Planning"

Food is pervasive in our society. In the 1960s, the average supermarket stocked about 6,000 items. Today, supermarkets stock more than 30,000 items. Take an item as simple as salad dressing. Almost 40 linear feet of shelf space is devoted to salad dressing encompassing all the different brands and flavors.

Our food society extends way beyond the supermarket. We have dedicated cable networks that are devoted solely to food. We have food magazines. Every day, hundreds of articles appear in the popular media with new recipes. The Internet and bloggers add to the food media overload. With this preponderance of food products, information, and services, it's fair to say that Americans love food.

Fitness and weight-loss experts have suggested that this food saturation has led to obesity. Scientists have suggested that large increases in obesity have paralleled the introduction of high-fat, energy-dense foods. The problem is that this simplistic equation does not necessarily hold true. Food trends have indicated that the American diet actually consists of less fat. This has given rise to the carbohydrate explanation, which says that the large increases in obesity began with the introduction of low-fat foods.

As people substituted high-carbohydrate foods for high-fat foods, there was little reduction in total caloric intake. And, in fact, people assumed that low-fat food was always healthier, even though nutritionists have pointed out that many of the low-fat foods may actually be higher in calories than their high-fat counterparts.

Since fat plays an important role in appetite regulation, low-fat diets may have interfered with the body's natural appetite controls. The result is that we are hungrier and therefore consume more food.

Just as there are many brands of salad dressing in our supermarkets today, there are many reasons why people eat, many of which have nothing to do with survival. Every culture of the world has rituals that are connected to food. It is used in wedding and holiday celebrations, given as gifts, shared in community gardens, and celebrated at harvest time. It is eaten on feast days and avoided on fasting days. Depending on how it is used, food can harm us or heal us.

If you look at our Paleolithic ancestor as the model, the striking difference is that today we have an abundance of food all the time, whereas our Paleolithic ancestors did not. As you have seen, having an abundance of food all the time disrupts the functional rhythms that control appetite, energy, and the ability to manufacture protein.

It is obvious that the "abundant food all the time" paradigm is not going to change within the foreseeable future. The government and the food industry have a vested interest in maintaining the status quo. Even the health food industry deserves a proportional share of the blame. Healthy food consumed without regard to the body's natural functional rhythm can contribute to our collective lack of fitness, just as much as the worst kind of fast food.

We are not going to suggest that you change the reasons why you eat. That would be a monumental task. However, we would like to introduce a component that we call the "ampersand connection." The ampersand connection focuses on one word—functionality. Timing the eating as well as the composition of your meals to your body's natural functional rhythm is the first step to living a fitness lifestyle. (Keep in mind that image of the boulder in the introduction.) When you ignore your body's functional rhythm, it is like trying to push a large boulder up the fitness summit. It is very difficult. On the other hand, when you take advantage of your body's natural functional rhythm it is like pushing the boulder downhill.

So what does this all have to do with the ampersand connection? The ampersand connection requires that you do not suddenly redefine your attitude toward food. If you love food and you eat for satisfaction, any diet that suggests that you give up the foods that provide this satisfaction will not be right for you. However, it is not difficult to eat satisfying foods that you love in the context of the body's natural functional rhythm. This means that regardless of where you shop, you will be able to select foods that are both satisfying and functional. If you like fast food, there are times when the best functional foods are higher protein/higher fat.

The key is to ensure that your food selections are matched to the body's natural functional rhythms. When the Activity Interval is open, a high-fat, high-protein fast-food entrée will not satisfy the functional needs of your body. In the evening, when the protein turnover interval is greatest, and dinner has been shown to be the least satiating meal of the day, protein and fat serve an important functional role.

Of course, synchronizing your body's macronutrient consumption with its functional rhythm is not a free ticket to eat as much as you want. Your total calories consumed have to be in balance with your total calories expended. But this becomes easier since the body's natural functional rhythm provides effective appetite control and highly efficient conversion of food into energy.

Resolution #5   "I Will Only Participate in Exercise Activities that Are Fun and Enjoyable"

Young children do not exercise. Although this is changing, the majority of them manage to stay quite lean. They don't exercise, but they do play. Scientists have measured the amount of calories burned by children playing. It is quite considerable, as any adult who is trying to keep up with a three- or four-year-old eight hours a day with tell you. It is exhausting. There is an object lesson here that gets ignored by many fitness and weight-loss experts. Everyone will agree that activity is essential, and you have certainly seen that your body's hardwiring only works when certain minimum levels of activity occur each day.

Paleolithic man certainly never thought about exercise, any more than he thought about keeping his heart beating. It was a natural consequence of his life and essential for survival. Our society is more complex. Opportunities for activity are decreasing, particularly in this country. Therefore, it is necessary that you create new opportunities to maintain your body's minimum level of activity.

Here is a typical scenario. An overweight person goes to a healthcare professional or enrolls in an Internet diet program. The individual receives a diet plan that ignores the body's functional rhythm and an activity program that ignores his or her personal likes. We can't count how many times we have seen professionals publish articles on weight loss. Most of the articles focus on nutrition and total calories consumed, and then, as an afterthought, there is a mandatory section on increasing daily activity as an essential part of a weight-loss regimen.

The number one activity recommended is walking. Walking is a great activity. It's low intensity and can be done almost anywhere and by anyone. The problem is that some people hate walking. If they are forced into an activity that they dislike from the start, compliance will be low, and they will eventually drop out of the program, which is a very familiar refrain describing weight-loss efforts in our current culture.

We recently completed a large attitudinal study among 2,800 serious endurance athletes. These athletes were primarily runners, cyclists, and triathletes. They did not represent the population norm. They exercised seriously three or more times a week. For most of the participants, their weights only fluctuated 5 to 10 pounds during the year. I am sure you are asking, "What could these individuals tell me when I am 30 pounds over-weight, have love handles, and get out of breath walking up steps?"

A major part of this study was to determine why these individuals exer-cise. They had many responses to choose from. They could have selected health, longevity, competition, or personal appearance, to name a few, but the number one reason given throughout all age groups and genders was *enjoyment*. These individuals enjoy exercise.

And that, in a nutshell, describes what is wrong with the "start a walk-ing program" approach to activity participation. If you don't enjoy walking, you won't do it. The enjoyment component is essential to long-term com-pliance and the ability to incorporate activity into your daily regimen.

SUMMARY

Although the Hardwired Fitness Program can help you become fit, it will not work unless you are committed mentally and emotionally. Unlike New Year's fitness resolutions, which are broken soon after they are made, suc-cess with the Hardwired Fitness Program demands that you make the fol-lowing lifestyle resolutions:

Resolution #1: "I will never diet again."

Resolution #2: "I will be patient."

Resolution #3: "I will take advantage of every opportunity to increase my daily lifestyle activity."

Resolution #4: "I will add functionality to my meal planning."

Resolution #5: "I will only participate in exercise activities that are fun and enjoyable."

PART TWO

The Hardwired Fitness Program

B y now it should be obvious that unless you restore your body's natural metabolic rhythm it will be extremely difficult—if not impossible—to achieve your fitness goals. A finely tuned engine runs better, has more power, and is more fuel-efficient. The Hardwired Fitness Program is a 24-week plan consisting of three phases:

- Phase One (Chapter 8) shows you how to restore your body's natural metabolic rhythm. In this 2-week phase, you will make adjustments to reach your threshold level of activity and sleep and implement the core principles of Functional Eating.

- Phase Two (Chapter 9) focuses on how to switch your body into fitness mode. In this 4-week phase, you will increase your daily caloric expenditure through changes in lifestyle activity and exercise, along with minor modifications to your Functional Eating Plan.

- Phase Three (Chapter 10) gets you into the red zone. Here is when you'll really start to see the results of resyncing your circuitry and making small adaptations that will optimize your fitness program. During weeks 7 through 24, you will build on the changes you made in Phases One and Two and periodically assess your fitness status to gauge your progress.

To make the program extremely easy to implement, we have developed a Hardwired Tool Kit. The tool kit found in Chapter 11 provides all the resources you need to be successful. We will refer you to it often throughout the program. If you follow the Hardwire Fitness Program, in just 24 weeks you will have painlessly instituted permanent lifestyle changes, resulting in improved weight control, greater lean body mass, and increased energy.

CHAPTER 8

Phase One:
Restore Your Natural
Metabolic Rhythm

Restoring your body's natural metabolic rhythm is the prerequisite first step to achieving your fitness goals. This is easier than you might imagine. A remarkable characteristic of the body is its ability to resynchronize its circuitry when the conditions are right. The four essential conditions that must be satisfied are:

1. Your daily level of activity must meet your threshold level.

2. Your daily sleep time must meet your threshold level.

3. Your mealtimes must be synchronized to the body's natural metabolic rhythm.

4. The nutrient composition of your meals must be matched to the metabolic activity of each functional interval. In other words, you must eat the right foods at the right time.

1. REACHING YOUR THRESHOLD LEVEL OF ACTIVITY

Your threshold level of activity is the minimum amount of energy you must expend each day through a combination of lifestyle activities and exercise to keep your fitness circuits in balance. The importance of reaching this threshold level cannot be overemphasized. In case you still need convincing, consider the findings from a recent study in which non-exercising healthy individuals reduced their daily activity by 80 percent, or significantly below their threshold level. The researchers then measured a number of fitness and metabolic parameters. The results were sobering to say the least: After just two weeks, the researchers found an increase in insulin resistance, which is associated with obesity and type 2 diabetes; a 7 percent decrease in cardiovascular fitness; and almost a 3 percent decrease in lean body mass.

Failure to reach your daily threshold level is a major obstacle to fitness and permanent weight loss. Ideally, exercise should be an essential element of the energy expenditure equation. Unfortunately, for most people it is not. Even individuals who exercise regularly may only do it three to four times a week. A fundamental principle in resyncing the fitness circuits is recognizing that the body operates on a 24-hour cycle. You must reach your threshold level of activity each and every day. For the vast majority of people who are out of shape, this means increasing their daily energy expenditure through lifestyle activities. This is not to minimize the importance of exercise; as you will see in Phase Two, exercise is an integral part of becoming fit. However, your initial goal should be to attain your threshold level by increasing or modifying your lifestyle activities.

Reaching your threshold level involves (1) calculating what is the minimum level based on your gender and weight, (2) completing a Personal Energy Inventory, (3) and making modifications in your lifestyle activity if your Personal Energy Inventory reveals that you are below your minimum threshold level. The following sections walk you through the details. Page 170 in the Hardwired Tool Kit contains a worksheet so you can record and analyze your results.

CALCULATE YOUR MINIMUM THRESHOLD LEVEL

There is an easy way to determine your minimum threshold level. Table 8.1 gives the threshold activity constants for women and men over a wide range of weights.

Simply find your weight under the appropriate table and multiply it by the constant provided. Record your results on the worksheet. For example, a woman weighing 150 pounds would have a threshold level of 705 calories (150 lbs × 4.7) per day; a man weighing 200 pounds would have a daily threshold activity level of 988 calories (200 lbs × 4.8). These individuals

| Table 8.1. Threshold Activity Level by Gender | | | |
| Women | | Men | |
Weight	Multiplier	Weight	Multiplier
Below 120	5.4	Below 120	6.0
120–145	5.2	121–145	5.8
146–165	4.7	146–175	5.2
166–190	4.4	176–200	4.9
191–230	4.0	201–230	4.8
Above 230	3.8	Above 230	4.7

would have to expend 705 and 988 calories per day, respectively, through their lifestyle activities to reach their threshold level. Assuming that the average day for most adults is 16 hours, this doesn't seem like a particularly high bar, but unfortunately most people don't reach it.

COMPLETE A PERSONAL ENERGY INVENTORY

Once you have calculated your threshold level of activity, the next step is to do a detailed activity inventory of your day to determine if you are reaching your daily threshold level. This step is critical. Creating a Personal Energy Inventory may seem complicated but here too it's really quite easy to do. Basically, you will reconstruct your daily waking activities for an average day. Refer to the list of common activities beginning on page 172 of the tool kit. Each activity has specific calorie expenditures per pound per minute of activity. It is not necessary nor is it practical to do a minute-by-minute inventory. Think of your activities in 15- or 30-minute increments. Many similar activities have the same caloric expenditure. If your lifestyle activity is not listed, select one that is comparable and use that energy value in determining your total daily energy expenditure.

After you identify each of your daily activities, use the worksheet on page 171 to record the activity, along with the net calories expended and the time you spent on each activity. This exercise tells you how much energy you expend in an average day in lifestyle- and occupational-related activities.

Next compare the total calories you expend through all of your lifestyle activities to the minimum threshold activity level. Some of you will find, after completing your inventory, you are exceeding your threshold level, which is great. Others will find that a few minor adjustments will get you to the needed level. Unfortunately for others, for whom net-zero activities represent a large segment of the day, getting yourselves to move more will require discipline. To reach that goal you have to look at how much of your day consists of net zero activities.

"Net-Zero" Activities

Inactivity is an unfortunate byproduct of modern life. Many of us work at a desk, we commute long hours to work, and when we come home we finish dinner and spend time before bed either surfing the Internet or watching TV. Table 8.2 describes many of the familiar activities that make up the average day, and here is the problem: most of these sedentary activities can be accurately called "net-zero" activities. In other words, activities that produce no or almost no additional energy expenditure over your resting level, or the amount of calories you burn when you are sleeping. Net-zero activities provide no benefit in helping you reach your threshold level. In fact, a preponderance of net-zero activities serves as a principal obstacle to optimizing the functioning of your fitness circuits.

LIFESTYLE ACTIVITY SUBSTITUTION

The good news, however, is that during the course of the day you have multiple occasions to increase your lifestyle activity, thereby helping you achieve your threshold level. Because your lifestyle activities are spread across your waking hours, small increases can get you to your threshold level. The easiest way to do this is through activity substitution; in other words, replace in whole or in part low-energy expenditure activities with higher energy expenditure activities. Table 8.2 also lists activities that are net positive. Simply substituting activities is painless and does not require a major change in your daily routine.

Table 8.2. Activity Substitution

NET-ZERO ACTIVITIES	Net Calories Expended (calories/lb body weight/ minute activity)
Napping	0
Lying quietly, doing nothing, lying in bed awake, listening to music	0
Lying quietly, watching television	0
Meditating	0
Reclining and reading	0
Reclining and talking, or talking on the phone	0
Reclining and writing	0
Riding in a car	0
Sitting quietly and watching television	0
Sitting and reading, book, newspaper, etc.	0.002
Sitting and talking or talking on the phone	0.004

HIGHER CALORIE EXPENDITURE ACTIVITIES	Net Calories Expended (calories/lb body weight/ minute activity)
Standing during miscellaneous activities	0.008
Walking on job, less than 2.0 mph, slowly	0.008
Cooking or food preparation and standing or sitting	0.008
Food shopping with or without a grocery cart, standing or walking	0.010
Multiple household tasks light effort	0.011
Putting away groceries (e.g., carrying groceries)	0.011
Washing dishes; clearing dishes from table	0.011
Sitting while playing with children	0.011
Walking, 2.5 mph, downhill	0.014
Child care: standing while dressing, bathing	0.015
Walking, 2.5 mph, firm surface	0.015
Walking, 3.0 mph, moderate pace, firm level surface	0.017

You would be surprised at how many opportunities you have during the day to increase your lifestyle activity. It could be as easy as:

- Parking your car in a space farthest from work

- Taking the stairs instead of the escalator or elevator

- Walking to lunch rather than driving

- Standing instead of sitting while talking on the phone or even better, pace when on the phone

- Cutting your lunch short by 15 minutes to take a short walk before returning to work

- Having a walk-and-talk meeting with a coworker rather than an office meeting

- Washing and drying dishes rather than using the dishwasher

The considerable amount of time that most of us spend sitting provides us with numerous opportunities to convert sitting into a net-positive activity. Completing a Personal Energy Inventory and making the necessary adjustments in your daily activities is not a paper exercise. You need to put your new activity plan into practice.

The inset on page 117 describes how Mary G. conducted a Personal Energy Inventory and what lifestyle modifications she made after discovering she was below her threshold level by 102 calories.

2. REACHING YOUR THRESHOLD LEVEL OF SLEEP

Lack of adequate sleep can play havoc with normal functioning of the fitness circuits. When nightly sleep falls below a threshold level it causes a major disruption in the working efficiency of the four fitness circuits. Sleep time is the only factor that disrupts the natural functioning of all four fitness circuits. The relationships between sleep debt and weight gain, increased appetite, decreased lean body mass, and lower energy levels have been well documented. Although there is individual variation on what represents the ideal amount of sleep time, studies show that, on average,

Mary G.'s Personal Energy Inventory

Mary G. is 5 feet 7 inches tall and weighs 150 pounds. She works for an insurance company, commutes to work by car, and has two boys ages 8 and 12. Using Table 8.1, she calculated that her Threshold Activity Level is 705 calories per day. Mary used the list of common activities found in the in the Hardwired Tool Kit to determine the calorie expenditure for each of her daily leisure and occupational activities. She approximated the amount of time she spent in each activity and recorded this information on the worksheet. Mary then multiplied her weight times the calorie expenditure for each activity, times the minutes she spent on each activity. For example, the total number of calories per day that she spent working at her desk job was 252 calories (150 lbs × 0.004 × 420 minutes). She did this for each of the activities and computed the calories she burns from her lifestyle activities at 603 calories per day, which put her 102 calories below her threshold level (see below).

Table 8.3. Personal Energy Inventory of Lifestyle Activities *Before* Adjustments

Activity	A. Weight (pounds)	B. Net Calories Expended	C. Time (minutes)	A x B x C Total Calories Expended
Typing on a computer	150	0.004	420	252
Sitting reading	150	0.000	55	0
Driving	150	0.007	120	126
Multiple household tasks	150	0.011	75	124
Cooking	150	0.001	60	9
Food shopping	150	0.009	35	47
Talking on the phone	150	0.004	75	45
Watching TV	150	0.000	120	0
Total			960	603

As with most of us, however, Mary's Personal Energy Inventory included three net-zero activities—reading, watching TV, and talking on the phone while sitting. Mary made the following adjustments in her daily lifestyle. Whenever she was talking on the phone she stood; she reduced the time that she spent watching TV; and she added 40 minutes of walking to her day by doing a 20-minute walk after lunch, taking the stairs instead of the elevator, and parking her car at a more distant lot. These three changes raised her lifestyle activity to 736 calories per day, putting her above her needed threshold level (see below).

Table 8.4. Personal Energy Inventory of Lifestyle Activities *After* Adjustments

Activity	A. Weight (pounds)	B. Net Calories Expended	C. Time (minutes)	A x B x C Total Calories Expended
Typing on a computer	150	0.004	420	252
Sitting reading	150	0.000	55	0
Driving	150	0.007	120	126
Multiple household tasks	150	0.011	75	124
Cooking	150	0.001	60	9
Food shopping	150	0.009	35	47
Standing talking on the phone	150	0.007	75	84
Watching TV	150	0.000	80	0
Walking for pleasure	150	0.019	40	112
Total			960	736

when you get less than seven and a half hours per night, it results in subtle but recognizable changes in how your fitness circuits operate. The problem is modern lifestyles often make it difficult to regularly get the sleep your circuits need and even if you get to bed to insure the proper amount of sleep, the stress of the day's activities often can keep you awake.

A GOOD NIGHT'S SLEEP

You can't sleep your way to fitness but lack of sleep will make the path to fitness much more difficult to travel. Fortunately, there are a number of excellent strategies to help you get the sleep you need. Here are a few:

Stay on schedule. Try to go to bed and get up at about the same time every day, even on the weekends. This helps reinforce your circadian sleep-wake cycle.

Program your body for bed. Do the same things each night to tell your body it's time to wind down. This may include taking a warm bath or shower, reading a book, or listening to soothing music. Relaxing activities done with lowered lights can help.

Create a sleep environment. Adjust the lighting, temperature, humidity and noise level to your preferences. Make your bedroom dark, cool, quiet, and comfortable. If you can't make your bedroom totally dark, wear an eye mask when you sleep. If too much quiet is a problem, try running a fan or using a device that generates sounds like the ocean waves breaking or rain falling that may help people who are sound-sensitive to sleep.

Avoid stimulants in the evening. Alcohol can disrupt normal sleeping patterns; the same holds true for caffeine.

Don't eat or drink large amounts before bedtime. Make sure you eat dinner no later than 8:00 P.M. We will also discuss in the next section the ideal nutrition during the Sleep Interval. If you're prone to heartburn, avoid spicy or fatty foods. Limit how much you drink before bed. Too much liquid can cause you to wake up repeatedly during the night for trips to the bathroom.

Sleep primarily at night. Daytime naps may steal hours from nighttime slumber. Limit daytime sleep to about a half hour and make it during mid-afternoon.

Go to bed when you're tired and turn out the lights. To help fall asleep and put worries out of your mind, try one of the following:

* Close your eyes and try taking deep, slow breaths; make each breath even deeper than the last.

- Close your eyes and imagine a place or activity that is calming and peaceful for you. Concentrate on how relaxed this place or activity makes you feel.

- Starting at your toes, tense all the muscles as tightly as you can, then completely relax. Work your way up from your feet to the top of your head.

If you don't fall asleep within 15 to 20 minutes, get up and do something else. Go back to bed when you're tired. Don't agonize over falling asleep. The stress will only prevent sleep.

Exercise regularly—but not right before bedtime. Physical activity, especially aerobic exercise, can help you fall asleep faster and make your sleep more restful.

Choose a comfortable mattress and pillow. Features of a good bed are subjective and differ for each person. But make sure you have a bed that's comfortable.

For many people reorganizing their sleep schedule, especially in two weeks, so that they can reach their threshold level of sleep may not be realistic. If this is your case, don't despair. Even if you don't reach the ideal level of seven and a half hours, your fitness efforts will not be sabotaged. Nevertheless, continue making the appropriate adjustment in your schedule so you do reach this level. Just remember your goal is to maximize the efficiency of your fitness circuits. An engine running at 85 percent efficiency performs better than one running at 70 percent. Each modification, including sleep time, made in Phase One gets you closer to your goal.

3. SYNCHRONIZE YOUR EATING TO YOUR BODY'S NATURAL METABOLIC RHYTHM

The body's 24-hour circadian cycle is divided into four distinct functional intervals. Taking advantage of the functional intervals—Restoration, Activity, Rebuilding, and Sleep—gives you a valuable tool to achieve your fitness goals. What's more, you don't have to change when you eat because the timing of the four functional intervals closely parallels our traditional meal segmentation of breakfast in the morning, lunch at midday, and dinner in the early evening.

THE FOUR FUNCTIONAL INTERVALS

Breakfast (Restoration 7:00 A.M.–9:00 A.M.)

Breakfast plays a pivotal role in maintaining the body's 24-hour natural rhythm. This meal is responsible for reducing the build up of physiological stress that naturally occurs in your body as a consequence of going without food while you sleep. The restoration meal also must recharge your energy circuits in preparation for the mental and physical activities of the day. For these reasons, carbohydrate (the body's main source of rapid energy) is a key macronutrient to consume during this interval. Although Functional Eating does not normally place a priority on a specific interval, the restoration meal is unique in that its influence is felt throughout the entire day. For example, people who eat breakfast are less hungry over the course of the day than breakfast skippers. If you don't normally wake up hungry, wait an hour or so for your appetite to kick in but never skip breakfast. It's that important. And always make sure to eat healthy forms of carbohydrate and the recommended number of calories based on your customized meal plan.

Lunch (Activity 9:00 A.M.–5:00 P.M.)

The Activity Interval represents the largest functional segment of the day—at least eight hours for most people. The body is programmed to be active during the daylight hours. As a result, during this interval the energy circuits are in their most active state. Your body will perform best by consuming high carbohydrate foods during this interval since your brain relies predominantly on carbohydrates for energy and muscles convert carbohydrates into energy more efficiently than protein or fat. During the late afternoon, for most of us there is a marked decline in energy expenditure. Thus, the latter stages of the Activity Interval represent an ideal time to consume a nutritious supplement that is high in macronutrients, such as fat and protein. These macronutrients are more satiating than carbohydrates. By doing so, you extend the feeling of fullness and avoid late-afternoon hunger cravings that are so common.

Dinner (Rebuilding 5:00 P.M.—8:00 P.M.)

The Rebuilding Interval between 5:00 P.M. and 8:00 P.M. is the time when the circuit responsible for rebuilding and restoring protein is most active. Just as carbohydrate is the most efficient macronutrient to consume during the Activity Interval, protein is the most efficient macronutrient to be consumed during the Rebuilding Interval. Foods high in protein are more easily converted into muscle protein. The protein you eat during this interval also provides another practical benefit because protein is a very satiating macronutrient. Meals consumed later in the day have been shown to be less satisfying. This may explain why overweight people shift their daily caloric consumption into the evening hours. Researchers have found marked differences between normal weight and overweight individuals in what time of day they ate. Overweight individuals were two to three times more likely to consume a higher proportion of their daily calories after their evening meal compared with normal weight individuals. In fact, overweight individuals consumed up to 25 percent of their daily calories after their evening meal. To help control hunger, the Rebuilding Interval is also an ideal time to consume the fats you need. Fats, especially healthy or unsaturated fats (discussed later), provide a very strong satiety or fullness effect. Seafood, olive oil, soybeans, and walnuts are a great source of healthy fats.

Anti-Stress Supplement (Sleep 11:00 P.M.—7:00 A.M.)

During the Sleep Interval the body is breaking down nutrients to maintain essential cellular function. This is a normal physiological process, which unfortunately involves the breakdown of muscle protein. You don't necessarily want to stop this process but it is certainly beneficial to minimize the amount of protein that is broken down. Consuming a high-protein beverage or food such as cottage cheese or turkey that won't interfere with your sleep can play an important role in modulating the effects of this physiological stress.

YOU CAN'T HAVE IT NOW

We live in a world where instant gratification rules. Food, both healthful and unhealthful, is available whenever we crave it. Our desire for instant gratification is in conflict with how the body's fitness circuitry works. The fitness circuits use nutrition most efficiently and effectively when our mealtimes are synchronized to the body's natural metabolic rhythm.

The functional intervals described in this section are not just suggestions on when and what to eat. A fundamental principle of the Hardwire Fitness Program is that you cannot ignore the specific timing and nutritional needs of each functional interval. The master clock that controls your body's metabolic rhythms evolved over millions of years. It is naive and unrealistic to think you can reset it at will just because you can buy a pizza at 11:00 P.M.

4. EATING THE RIGHT FOODS AT THE RIGHT TIME

Although the body has the ability to convert carbohydrates, proteins, and fats from one form to another, each of these three macronutrients has principle metabolic functions:

- Proteins are used to make up cell structure, form enzymes, and repair and rebuild muscle protein. They provide the energy necessary to drive all metabolic reactions in the body and to help release hormones, peptides, and neurotransmitters (brain chemicals) that suppress appetite. Proteins are the most satiating of the macronutrients.

- Carbohydrates are used for rapid energy. Their bulk activates nerves in the stomach that tell the brain to stop eating. Carbohydrates also play an important role in preventing and reducing the buildup of stress hormones such as cortisol, which in turn impacts appetite fat utilization and body composition.

- Fats are used for sustained energy and appetite suppression. They slow down digestion, postponing the time before the stomach senses hunger and begins signaling the brain to stimulate appetite again.

It stands to reason that if the body's functions change in a predictable way over a 24-hour period, then the macronutrient composition of your meals should change accordingly. The logic of synchronizing what you eat to your body's natural functional rhythm seems irrefutable, yet this basic concept is ignored by every popular eating plan, including primal diets such as the Paleolithic or caveman diet and those recommended by prestigious organizations such as the American Heart Association (AHA). The AHA diet is a high-carbohydrate, low-fat eating plan; the Paleolithic diet is a low-carbohydrate, high-protein eating plan. Although these two popular diets differ widely in their recommended macronutrient composition, both are similar in that they impose macronutrient rigidity over the day. As shown in Figures 8.1a, 8.1b, and 8.1c, this lack of synchrony could not be more evident when one compares these two eating plans with the macronutrient requirements based on the body's natural metabolic rhythm. This lack of synchrony also explains why in spite of the diets' substantial differences in carbohydrate, protein, and fat percentages, they and other popular diets all deliver roughly the same lack of results long-term.

Now compare the nutrient requirements of the Hardwired Fitness Program (Figure 8.2) with how the body works (Figure in 8.1a). In spite of the enormous body of supporting science conducted over the past 50 years, the Hardwired Fitness Program is the first eating plan that is based on the body's metabolic rhythm and changing macronutrient needs.

The impact of synchronizing what you eat to the body's natural functional intervals is considerable. Earlier in the book we described a study illustrating the importance of nutrient timing, particularly after exercising. The results showed that there were significant benefits in terms of replenishing energy stores and repairing and rebuilding muscle protein if a nutritional beverage was consumed immediately after exercise. However, the magnitude of the recovery response was doubly impacted by the nutrient composition of the beverage. A beverage containing a mixture of protein and carbohydrate stimulated the manufacture of protein 38 percent more than one containing just protein and 100 percent more than a beverage containing just carbohydrate.

If you synchronize the timing of your meals to the body's functional intervals, you gain a metabolic advantage. However, if you combine the

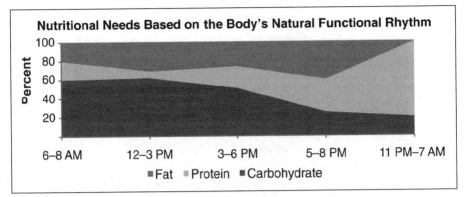

Figure 8.1a. Daily macronutrient composition based on the body's natural functional rhythm.

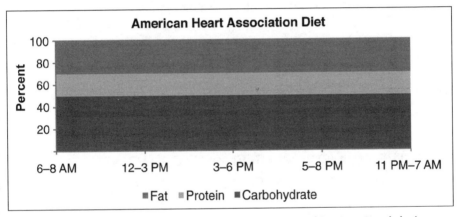

Figure 8.1b. Daily macronutrient composition based on American Heart Association's recommendations.

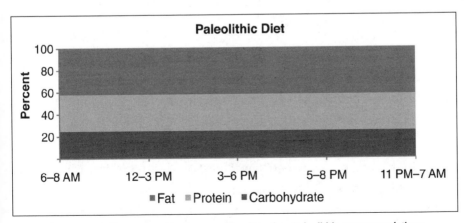

Figure 8.1c. Daily macronutrient composition based on Paleolithic recommendations.

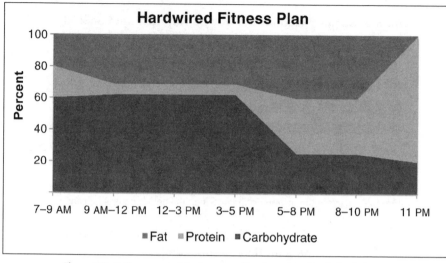

Figure 8.2. Daily macronutrient composition based on Hardwired Fitness eating plan recommendations.

timing of your meals with the right combination of nutrients, it will produce a positive synergistic effect on your metabolism.

THE FIVE PRINCIPLES OF FUNCTIONAL EATING

Functional Eating is not a complicated process. All you have to do is follow these five simple principles.

1. Eat high-carbohydrate foods between 7:00 A.M. and 1:00 P.M. (during the Restoration and Activity Intervals) to ensure that the muscles and brain have sufficient energy.

2. Decrease consumption of carbohydrate foods dramatically throughout the afternoon and evening.

3. Consume 55 percent of your daily calories by 1:00 P.M. to parallel the body's energy needs. In other words, eat less after 1:00 P.M. but eat foods that are more satiating.

4. Eat high-protein foods between 5:00 P.M. and 8:00 P.M. (during the Rebuilding Interval). The protein turnover circuit is most active during this period because it is not competing with the pathways responsible for generating energy.

5. Keep fat intake to a minimum in the morning and throughout most of the day, but increase its intake in the evening. Consumption of specific fats plays an important role in modulating appetite; these same fats are also the healthiest fats to consume. Since dinner has been shown to be the least satisfying or satiating meal of the day, this strategy helps keep you full in the period between dinner and bedtime.

Figure 8.3 shows how this macronutrient breakdown is allocated over the four functional intervals.

If you are extremely fit and have a high level of physical activity during the day, most eating plans will help you maintain your fitness level. Although the principles in the Hardwired Fitness Plan will help fit people get to the next level, this program is primarily directed to individuals who are not in shape. They need every metabolic advantage possible. Timing your meals to the body's functional intervals and changing your meal composition to optimize metabolic activity enables the fitness circuitry to operate at peak efficiency.

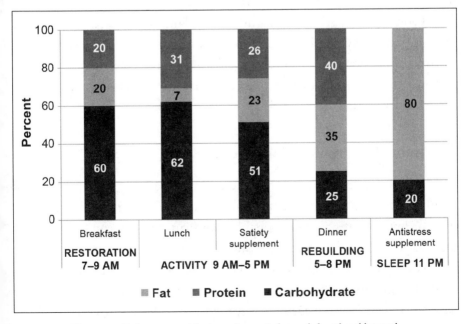

Figure 8.3. Daily macronutrient requirements for each functional interval.

How Our Paleolithic Ancestors Stayed Fit

An obvious question is how could our Paleolithic ancestors maintain their high level of fitness since it would have been most difficult for them to implement the principles of Functional Eating? The answer is simple. The daily lifestyle activity of our Paleolithic ancestors was sufficiently high that it compensated for a less-than-ideal diet. One remarkable attribute of the body's fitness circuitry is its ability to function normally over a wide range of conditions. The best example of how high activity can trump poor nutrition is seen in young athletes. They can eat almost anything and still maintain a very high level of fitness. Once their activity level drops, the circuitry dysfunction becomes very apparent as they rapidly lose their high level of fitness. Most of us are not athletes. We need an edge. The genetic adaptations in our DNA give us an edge if we take advantage of it.

CREATING A FUNCTIONAL EATING PLAN

An effective hook of many popular diets and eating plans is that you don't have worry about calories. The more unscrupulous ones even claim you can eat all you want and still lose weight. These plans imply that somehow they have found a way to alter the basic laws of thermodynamics. In other words, calories consumed in excess of what you burn simply disappear. Anyone who has ever gone on one of these diets knows through personal experience that they don't work.

Determine Your Daily Caloric Needs

Although Functional Eating has the ability to change your life, it still requires attention to the fundamentals of thermodynamics. Thus, the first step for implementing a Functional Eating Plan is to determine how many calories you need to consume to ensure that your body is in energy balance. To do this, you must know your total daily caloric expenditure, which is the total of your threshold activity, plus your resting calorie expenditure. We have created an easy and accurate way for you to calculate your daily caloric expenditure.

To determine your resting caloric expenditure, find your weight in Table 8.5 and multiply your weight by the assigned constant. Likewise, to determine your minimum threshold activity level, find your weight in Table 8.6 and multiply it by the assigned constant. Add the two values. This number represents your daily caloric needs and becomes the basis of selecting an appropriate meal plan.

Table 8.5. Resting Caloric Expenditure

Women		Men	
Weight	Multiplier	Weight	Multiplier
Below 120	11.2	Below 120	12.2
120–130	10.5	120–135	11.7
131–150	9.8	136–160	10.9
151–175	9.1 = *1547*	161–185	10.3
176–210	8.4	186–210	9.8
211–230	7.8	211–230	9.3
Above 230	7.5	Above 230	9.0

Table 8.6. Minimum Threshold Activity Level Expenditure

Women		Men	
Weight	Multiplier	Weight	Multiplier
Below 120	5.5	Below 120	6.2
120–145	5.2	121–145	5.8
146–165	4.7	146–175	5.2
166–190	4.4 *748*	176–200	4.9
191–230	4.0	201–230	4.8
Above 230	3.8	Above 230	4.7

2295

For example, if you are a female who weighs 160 pounds your threshold activity expenditure is 752 calories per day (160 lbs × 4.7) and your resting calorie expenditure is 1,568 (160 × 9.8) calories per day. Your total daily caloric needs are 2,319 calories (752 calories + 1,567 calories). Your daily caloric consumption is based on this value.

Once you have identified your resting caloric expenditure, minimum threshold activity expenditure, and daily caloric needs, use the worksheet on page 170 to record the numbers.

Figure 8.4 shows how a diet of approximately 2,300 calories per day is allocated over the four functional intervals.

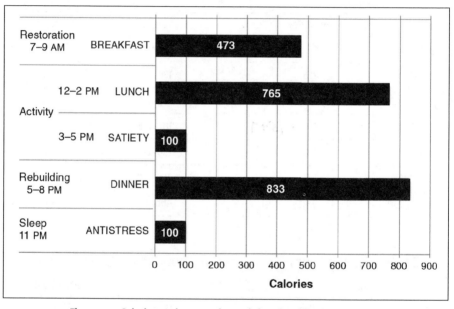

Figure 8.4. Calorie requirements for each functional interval based on a daily diet of 2,300 calories.

Choose Your Meal Plan

Once you determine your daily caloric needs, you'll need to select the meal plan that is closest to these needs. Until now, we have described Functional Eating in terms of calories and carbohydrate, protein, and fat composition. We realize, however, that you don't eat calories and macronutrients—you eat meals made with real foods. Food is a wonderful part of our lives. A focus on the functionality of what you eat does not necessarily mean you will be giving up on the satisfaction and pleasure that comes from eating a varied and delicious diet. To the contrary, a major problem with many of the popular eating plans is that they try to severely limit consumption of a major food group. By doing so, there is a corresponding decrease in the variety of food choices. This often leads to meal tedium, eating the same thing every day. Whereas, an eating plan based on function gives you a greater variety of choices.

Working with Brittany Crim, a registered dietician at the University of Texas, we have created nutritious meal plans based on different daily calorie requirements. The Hardwired Tool Kit offers meal plans for 1,800-, 2,000-, 2,300-, 2,500-, 2,800- and 3,000-calorie diets (see pages 177–189). Each of these plans gives you multiple food choices for every meal. All the meal plans are consistent with the principles of Functional Eating in terms of calories and macronutrient composition. Table 8.7 shows daily calorie allocation for meal plans ranging from 1,800 to 3,000 calories per day.

Table 8.7. Meal Calorie Recommendations for Different Daily Calorie Levels

Meal	1,800	2,000	2,300	2,500	2,800	3,000
Breakfast	368	420	473	525	578	630
Lunch	595	680	765	850	935	1,020
Satiety Supplement	100	100	100	100	100	100
Dinner	648	740	833	925	1,080	1,110
Anti-Stress Supplement	100	100	100	100	100	100

Select the meal plan that is closest to your daily caloric needs. You may have to make some minor adjustments. If your daily caloric requirements fall in between two of the calorie levels, select the lower one and simply add additional food to reach your recommended levels. For example, if your daily requirement is 2,150, use the 2,000-calorie plan and add a piece of fruit and a slice of bread to the lunch meal. With the Internet, there are also some excellent resources that will enable you to develop other food choices based on calories and the required macronutrient composition. We have listed some of these in the Resources section in the tool kit.

Strive as best you can to eat wholesome, nutritious foods. It is an unfortunate fact of life that today it is easier to eat unhealthily than healthily. Unhealthful foods are cheaper, more readily available, and more convenient. Since we can't create McFruits and McVegetables, we asked our dietitian how we could make eating well less complicated. See "Eating Healthier, Easier" on page 133 for some valuable suggestions.

ALL PROTEIN IS NOT EQUAL

Protein and other macronutrients are not equal in their ability to positively impact our fitness circuitry. Although protein is more effective in stimulating the manufacture of protein than carbohydrate or fat, there are major differences among proteins. For example, whey protein, because of its amino acid profile, is more effective in building new protein than protein from corn or wheat. We call whey a super-functional ingredient. Super-functional ingredients can have an additive impact on your fitness circuits and overall metabolism. Following are five super-functional ingredients that should be part of your daily diet. We will show you how these super-functional ingredients work and what foods are excellent sources for each of them. The Hardwired Tool Kit contains a more comprehensive listing of foods high in each super-functional ingredient. Whenever possible, include super-functional foods in your diet.

Branched-Chain Amino Acids

Proteins are composed of amino acids. Of the 21 amino acids, 10 are considered essential because the body cannot manufacture them; they must be consumed in your diet. Three of these essential amino acids—valine, leucine, and isoleucine—have a similar chemical structure and are called branched-chain amino acids or BCAAs.

BCAAs play an important role in activating the master switches that control the protein turnover and energy circuits. Leucine activates mTOR, the master switch that controls the protein turnover circuit. Studies have shown that when leucine is added to the diet it can enhance the building of muscle protein and lean body mass. For example, milk, a rich source of

Eating Healthier, Easier

1. **Be prepared!** Pick a day that you have more time and make sure to do your shopping and prepping of ingredients you may need throughout the week. It is also beneficial to take time to cook meals ahead of time. For example, make five breakfast tacos on Sunday and you will have them ready to go for Monday through Friday.

2. **Make lists.** Going to the grocery store without a list opens a window that will let "unhealthy" choices into your shopping cart. It also allows you to forget ingredients you need in order to prepare your food at home. Make a list of what you need ahead of time and stick to only what is on your list: this will save you money and time.

3. **Shop the perimeter of the grocery store.** The most whole and nutritious foods are located on the outer parts of the grocery store. The inner isles tend to have more highly processed and unhealthy food temptations that contain empty calories.

4. **Read labels.** When we are short on time, we often turn to convenience foods. If you find yourself in the situation where convenience foods are unavoidable, be sure you read your labels. Avoid foods high in saturated and/or trans fats as well as high in sodium.

5. **Have back-ups.** Keeping nutritious snacks such as almonds, granola, light popcorn in your desk or pantry can help you get through times of hunger when you don't have time to prepare a full meal.

6. **One and done!** When in social situations where food is being served in abundance, fill a small six-inch plate with your favorite choices and then be done for the rest of the event.

7. **Strive for 35.** Try to consume 35 grams of fiber each day. Choosing foods high in fiber will help you feel satisfied as well as pack your diet full of other essential nutrients. High-fiber foods tend to be lower in calories.

8. **Eat colorful.** The most colorful foods have the most nutrition. Fruits and vegetables are loaded with fiber and antioxidants, and are naturally low in calories. The more color, the more nutrition-packed the food is.

9. **Stay hydrated.** It is very common to misinterpret thirst for hunger. Making sure you are well hydrated can help you stay focused and avoid unnecessary grazing.

10. **Eat mindfully!** It is easy to over consume when you are in a rush or distracted. To eat mindfully means that you are aware of what you are putting into your body as well as how much you are putting in.

BCAAs, significantly improves protein synthesis compared with soy, which has a lower content of leucine. Every protein contains BCAAs. However, proteins found in certain foods such as beef, chicken eggs, and milk are naturally enriched with BCAAs (see also page 190). Eating foods high in BCAAs, particularly in the evening (Rebuilding Interval) when the protein turnover circuit is most active, will help improve body composition.

Long-Chain Fatty Acids

When you eat a high-fat meal, you feel full or satiated. However, not all fats are equally effective in blunting appetite. Researchers have shown that fatty acids that are between 10 and 18 carbons are most effective at blunting appetite. When you consume fats that contain long-chain fatty acids, they stimulate the release of the cholecystokinin or CCK, the body's primary feel-full protein. The released CCK produces a number of physiologic effects. It closes the valve between your stomach and GI tract, thereby slowing the movement of food from your stomach, which then begins to expand, giving you a feeling of fullness. It also travels to the appetite center in your brain that tells you to stop eating. Although CCK is one of the most important regulators of how full you feel, the body has additional ones that are also activated by long-chain fatty acids.

Foods high in long-chain fatty acids are even more satiating than protein. In the Functional Eating Plan, dinner should be high in protein and fat, particularly a healthful fat. High-protein foods provide the raw material to build muscle protein and at the same time help blunt appetite; foods high in healthy fats provide the body with this essential ingredient and are also more satiating. Consuming a dinner that is high in protein and healthy fat makes it less likely that you will be hungry and consume needless calories in the period after dinner and before going to bed.

Almonds, avocados, and olive oil are a few healthful foods that contain high levels of long-chain fatty acids; others are listed on page 190 in the tool kit.

B Vitamins

B vitamins play a special role in energy metabolism. Eight vitamins make up the B-vitamin complex: thiamine (B_1), riboflavin (B_2), niacin (B_3), pantothenic acid (B_5), pyridoxine (B_6), folate (B_9), cyanocobalamin (B_{12}), and biotin. As a group, these nutrients are vital coenzymes that aid in releasing energy from carbohydrates, fats, and proteins. Vitamin B_6 also assists in building proteins from amino acids.

Most of the B vitamins in the diet come attached to proteins in the foods you eat. A diet that contains high amounts of protein-rich foods such as meat, fish, poultry, dairy products, nuts, and beans provides plenty of B vitamins. Folate is found in the greatest abundance in green leafy vegetables and is the only member of the B-vitamin complex in which many people are deficient. You can ensure adequate folate intake by adding more green leafy vegetables to your diet and by taking a daily multivitamin with folic acid (the form found in supplements). Because of their role in energy metabolism foods containing B vitamins are particularly effective when consumed during the Restoration and Activity Intervals.

Soluble Fiber

Soluble fiber has a unique effect on the appetite circuit. Soluble fiber makes the appetite circuit work more efficiently. Soluble fibers have the ability to absorb water and swell, which help decrease appetite in two ways: First, when foods high in soluble fiber are consumed, they absorb water in the stomach, causing the stomach to expand. The uncomfortable feeling that results is often a signal to stop eating. Second, the expansion of the stomach activates a more important signal that helps control appetite. As the stomach expands, it stimulates the release of CCK. Thus, eating food that is high in fiber makes your feel-full mechanism turn on faster. Fruits, vegetables, and whole-grain foods are generally high in soluble fiber. For other good food sources, see page 190.

Because of its wide-ranging health benefits, foods high in soluble fiber should be consumed throughout all the functional intervals. However, soluble fiber is particularly valuable when consumed during the Restoration Interval (morning), the latter part of the Activity Interval (late afternoon), and the early part of the Rebuilding Interval (early evening).

CORE PRINCIPLES OF FUNCTIONAL EATING

Respect Your Body's Natural Rhythm

The body works on a 24-hour cycle. Every 24 hours your body resets its clock. You can't binge one day and starve yourself the next. You can't exercise vigorously on weekends and lead a sedentary life during the week. Nor can you run up a sleep debt during the week and expect to pay it off over the weekend by sleeping longer.

Reach Your Daily Threshold

The full benefits of Functional Eating only occur if you reach your threshold level of activity and sleep every day.

Don't Skip Meals or Add Meals

The Functional Eating Plan is specifically designed for you to consume three meals per day to dovetail with the three major functional intervals that occur during the day. The two 100-calorie supplements are to extend satiety and reduce the overnight buildup of stress during the Sleep Interval. Skipping meals creates two problems. First, it interferes with the normal function of your fitness circuits, and second, meal skipping results in greater calorie consumption. Studies have repeatedly shown that any calorie advantage gained when a meal is skipped is more than lost on the next meal, since hunger sensations are greater.

Never Skip or Skimp on Breakfast

All the points made about meal skipping apply to breakfast. However, breakfast provides benefits that extend throughout the day in terms of appetite modulation, and physical and mental energy levels.

Eat Carbohydrates Early in the Day

Consume carbohydrates through lunch and decrease carbohydrate consumption for the remainder of the day.

Eat Protein Later in the Day

Consume most of your daily protein requirements in the evening.

Calories Do Count

Although you are increasing the efficiency of your fitness circuitry by the timing and macronutrient composition of your meals, you simply cannot disregard calories. It is essential that you keep a caloric balance. Functional Eating will ensure that the food you eat will be more efficiently utilized. Once you disrupt the balance between calories expended and calories consumed, you lose the many benefits of Functional Eating.

SUMMARY

In Phase One, you establish four important conditions to restore your body's natural metabolic rhythm. This phase takes two weeks. In the first week, you focus on your daily energy expenditure. This involves determining your daily threshold level, completing a Personal Energy Inventory, and making the necessary adjustments in your lifestyle activities to ensure you reach your threshold level. In the second week, you focus on meal timing and meal composition. Meals are timed so they are synchronized to the body's four functional intervals and their nutrient composition is adjusted to optimize metabolic efficiency of the fitness circuits. Once you have restored your body's rhythm, you can then move on to the next phase— switching your body into fitness mode.

PHASE ONE: Restore Your Natural Metabolic Rhythm

Week	Activities
Week 1	• Calculate your threshold level of activity.
	• Complete a Personal Energy Inventory.
	• Make modifications in your lifestyle activities to ensure you reach your threshold level every day.
	• Make adjustments in your daily schedule to ensure you reach your threshold level of sleep.
Week 2	• Calculate your total daily calorie expenditure.
	• Implement a Functional Eating Plan.

CHAPTER 9

Phase Two:
Switch Your Body into Fitness Mode

In Phase Two, you're going to switch your body into fitness mode. This involves making a few simple modifications in your daily activity and eating patterns over the next four weeks. The changes you made in Phase One were designed to restore your body's natural rhythm. The small but important modifications you make in Phase Two are priming your body for change and are helping to establish healthful lifestyle and eating habits that will keep you fit for life. By making the changes gradually over four weeks your body has a chance to adapt.

The three key modifications that you will make are:

1. Increasing your daily threshold level of activity by 100 calories per day.

2. Adding 90 to 120 minutes of moderate exercise to your weekly schedule.

3. Decreasing your daily caloric intake by 200 calories.

1. INCREASING YOUR THRESHOLD LEVEL OF ACTIVITY

In Phase One, with small changes in your daily routine, you reached your threshold level of activity. During the first week of Phase Two, you are going to raise your lifestyle activity by 100 calories per day so that you will now be exceeding your threshold level of activity. The obvious question is, why not burn the extra calories by exercising. Exercise is a great way to help you raise your threshold level of activity—as long as you exercise every day. (Don't forget, your body works on a 24-hour cycle.) Yet the reality is, most people do not exercise every day. Therefore, we have found that the easiest way to increase your daily threshold level by 100 calories is to make a further modification in your lifestyle activity.

REVIEW YOUR PERSONAL ENERGY INVENTORY

To do this, review the Personal Energy Inventory that you created in week one. Even though you are now achieving your Threshold Activity Level, you will probably find there is still ample opportunity for converting net-zero activities to net-positive ones. Look for creative ways to move more throughout the day:

- Increase the length of time you walk; walking 40 minutes instead of 30 minutes increases your calorie expenditure by 20 percent.

- Increase the speed of your walk; increasing the pace from three miles per hour (20 minutes per mile) to four miles per hour (15 minutes per mile) increases your calorie expenditure by 43 percent.

- Carry a two-pound weight in each hand and swing your arms when you are walking; this not only increases your calorie burn by 20 percent, but also helps firm up your arm muscles since you now are doing hundreds of arm curls while you walk.

- Change your walking course so it has a slight grade; walking uphill increases caloric burn 15 percent compared to walking a flat course.

- Get up and visit office coworkers instead of emailing them.

- Work in your garden or manually wash your car.

- Bike to the store or use an exercise bike while watching TV.

Even time spent sitting is an opportunity to increase calorie burn, by incorporating a few stretching or resistance exercises. The Hardwired Tool Kit contains an easy exercise routine (page 191) you can do right at your desk. A small increase of 100 calories in your daily threshold activity will pay a big fitness dividend.

2. ADDING EXERCISE TO YOUR WEEKLY SCHEDULE

We are hardwired to be active throughout the day, but we are not hard-wired to exercise, which involves shorter bursts of activity on a voluntary basis. If we could mimic the daily routine of our Paleolithic ancestors, we would not have to set aside part of the day to exercise. Although your fitness circuits can be brought back into balance without a regular exercise program, improvements in body composition and overall fitness are going to occur more readily if you are willing to commit to three to four short exercise sessions a week.

Research over the past ten years has demonstrated that exercise plays an increasingly important role on the overall functioning of the fitness circuitry. Exercise, for example, increases the sensitivity of the fitness circuits. It stimulates the manufacture of new protein, improves appetite control, and increases energy while reducing stress, and much more.

Exercise Increases Fat Utilization and Decreases Fat Storage

The more you exercise, the more efficient your energy circuit functions. Exercise increases the body's sensitivity to insulin so it needs less insulin to control the energy circuit. Higher levels of insulin have a substantial impact on both body composition and fitness level. At rest and during exercise, higher insulin levels will inhibit the breakdown of fat for fuel. Without fat to burn, the body increases its reliance on carbohydrate to support its energy needs. This has three adverse effects: (1) it causes fatigue and rapid depletion of your carbohydrate stores, (2) it limits your ability to reduce body fat, and (3) it promotes greater storage of fat. Exercise, by reducing insulin levels, can prevent all three effects.

Exercise Increases Lean Body Mass

During periods of exercise when energy requirements are high, the protein turnover circuit is switched off. As you've learned, exercise increases the body's sensitivity to insulin. In the immediate interval postexercise, this is a major plus. Remember, insulin has multiple effects. It serves as a master switch to both the energy and protein turnover circuits. Immediately after exercise, insulin turns on the pathways that stimulate protein synthesis. This means that a higher percentage of nutrients you consume after exercise are converted to lean body tissue such as muscle and less to fat.

Increasing lean body mass not only improves your fitness level but also impacts weight management. Your resting calorie expenditure is a direct function of your muscle mass. A muscle cell requires seven times more energy each day than a fat cell. The fewer muscle cells—the lower your resting metabolic rate. Exercise, by increasing lean body mass, modifies this equation so it works in your favor. The greater your lean body mass, the higher your metabolic rate. Thus, exercise helps you burn more calories both when you are exercising and when you're not.

Exercise Helps Control Appetite

Interaction of the energy circuit with the appetite circuit occurs on two different levels. There is an immediate effect and a long-term effect that occurs with regular exercise. There is a misconception that an increase in physical activity always increases appetite and calorie consumption, which equals or is greater than the calories burned during physical exercise. This is not true.

Exercising regularly significantly impacts appetite. In Chapter 3, you saw that appetite is controlled by two different pathways: one pathway stimulates hunger, the other increases the feeling of fullness. Both pathways are under the control of specific proteins. Exercise inhibits the release of proteins that stimulate hunger and this inhibition can last for several hours after you stop exercising.

Researchers at East Carolina University found that moderate exercise led to a more sensible energy intake in overweight individuals. These findings reinforce the research we cited previously of Dr. Jean Mayer, who found that there was a tight coupling between daily energy expenditure and energy consumption, as long as energy expenditure was above a threshold level. When energy expenditure fell below the Threshold Activity

Level, there was an uncoupling between the energy and appetite circuits. This resulted in caloric consumption exceeding caloric expenditure and a gain in weight. Moreover, Mayer's results showed that the more one falls below his or her threshold activity level, the greater the imbalance between caloric expenditure and consumption.

It is true, however, that appetite is not always suppressed following exercise. Several studies have shown that exercise can make people hungrier resulting in an increase in calorie consumption after exercise. What is often not noted when these studies are cited is that the increase in food consumption following exercise was always less than the total amount of calories burned during exercise so that exercise still produces a caloric deficit.

An increase in appetite following exercise serves as an important survival function. It prevents the body from indefinitely expending fuel reserves in the event it is called upon to perform at a high level of physical exertion for a work-related task or during an emergency. If you do not replenish your energy stores on a daily basis, you will eventually compromise your body's ability to respond to a situation that requires a substantial physiological effort. And, over the long-term, you will become increasingly more lethargic.

Exercise Reduces Stress

Elevated levels of stress hormones like cortisol can increase your appetite, decrease your ability to utilize fat, and increase storage of abdominal fat. Exercise can be viewed as a form of stress. The secretion of cortisol and other stress-related hormones are critical physiological adaptations that permit you to engage in exercise. For example, these hormones are partially responsible for increasing heart rate and breathing, and for maintaining a steady supply of fuel to the working muscles during high energy-requiring activities such as exercise. However, the more you exercise, the fewer stress hormones are required to control these essential physiological functions. By modulating this increase, exercise helps minimize many of their detrimental effects.

EFFECTS OF EXERCISE ON HEALTH

A moderate amount of exercise weekly accomplishes two goals: it not only increases the efficiency of your fitness circuitry but also provides significant health benefits. You don't have to be an exercise fanatic to gain these benefits. Thirty minutes of exercise per day three to four days a week can have a profound effect on longevity, heart disease, type 2 diabetes, certain types of cancer, and bone health as shown below. The best part of exercise is that it is the gift that keeps on giving: the more you exercise in terms of time and frequency, the greater the benefits to your overall health.

Longevity

Individuals who exercise at a moderate level have a 20 to 50 percent lower risk of premature death than individuals who don't exercise. For people who are just starting an exercise program, the health benefits of exercise are greatest. The largest reduction in health risks occurs when one goes from being sedentary to being moderately physically active. For example, individuals who went from no exercise to exercising regularly over a five-year period were 44 percent less likely to die prematurely than those individuals who remained inactive.

Heart Disease

There is strong evidence that regular aerobic exercise protects against dying from cardiovascular and coronary heart disease. In a classic study Ralph Paffenbarger, a well-known researcher, found that college graduates who led a physically active lifestyle had a lower risk of death due to cardiovascular disease than alumni who did not engage in physical activities. This protective effect of exercise was seen with as little as one hour of brisk walking per week.

Type 2 Diabetes

Physically active individuals are much less likely to develop type 2 diabetes than very sedentary individuals. JoAnn Manson and her colleagues from

Harvard Medical School found that females who exercised at least once a week were 35 percent less likely to develop type 2 diabetes compared to women who did not exercise. These same researchers also found that men who exercised at least once a week had less body fat as well as a reduced incidence of type 2 diabetes than men who did not exercise. The protective effect of exercise is strongest in those individuals who have a family history of type 2 diabetes, obesity, and high blood pressure. Not only can exercise prevent the development of type 2 diabetes, but it also has been shown in the early stages of the disease to restore normal control of glucose. In some cases, type 2 diabetics who began an exercise program were able to stop taking oral medications and insulin injections.

Cancer

Recent research suggests that exercising regularly can reduce the risk of certain types of cancer including prostate, pancreatic, and melanoma, but particularly breast and colon cancers. Moderate exercise is associated with a 30 to 40 percent reduction in colon cancer risk in men and women, and a 20 to 30 percent reduction in breast cancer risk. This reduced risk was seen in women with and without a family history of breast cancer.

Bone Health

Weak or frail bones can compromise a person's quality of life and increase the risk of injury. A number of studies suggest that engaging in a regular exercise routine, particularly weight-bearing and resistance exercise, prevents bone loss associated with aging. In some cases, exercise was shown not only to slow bone loss but also to reverse bone loss by 1 to 2 percent per year.

Can Exercise Help You Lose Weight?

Although it has been proven that exercise provides many health benefits, from a practical perspective it is very difficult for exercise to produce weight loss. This almost seems to be a contrarian opinion. As weight loss has become the focal point of U.S. health policy, exercise has become a critical element in the recommendations. It is not surprising that the American College of Sports Medicine, of which we are both members, is extremely vocal in defending the benefits of exercise as part of a program to lose weight. We don't disagree that obesity represents our number one health problem; the key question is whether getting more people to exercise is the solution to obesity. The problem is that the amount of exercise found to effectively decrease weight may not be practical for most individuals. Experts in the weight-loss field maintain that 90 to 120 minutes of exercise per day is required for exercise to be effective for weight loss. This does not include changing and showering time, and is so unrealistic for the majority of Americans that we question how exercise alone can be recommended for weight loss. Moreover, studies have shown that exercise is no more effective than calorie restriction for weight loss.

Consider that in the last 20 years there has been an increase in the number of people who exercise regularly. At the same time, there has been an increase in the number of people who are overweight. What this says is that exercise cannot be solely viewed in the context of weight loss and that our health policy, by focusing primarily on losing weight rather than on fitness, has been a monumental failure.

If you focus on fitness, you will lose weight, improve body composition, and increase activity capacity. If you focus on weight loss, you may or may not be successful. Those who do succeed will be the individuals with the willpower and determination to keep pushing that large rock uphill. In terms of overall health outcomes, being fit is far more important than being lean and unfit, and regular exercise is an essential part of a fitness lifestyle.

COMMITING TO AN EXERCISE ROUTINE

If you are not presently exercising, it can be a daunting task to initiate a program. More commonly, you have probably started and stopped exercising multiple times in the past. Here are some questions you should ask yourself before beginning an exercise program. Start off right and you'll increase your chances of putting together an activity regimen you'll want to stick with.

What Should I Consider When Getting Started?

When beginning an exercise program, start slowly and then gradually build up. Plan your exercise routine weekly and try to select activities that you think you will enjoy doing. Schedule exercise time into your daily activities just like a business meeting. Set weekly and monthly goals, but be realistic in setting your goals. Keep a record of your exercise sessions and evaluate it weekly to see if you have met your goals. Following your goals can be a great motivator. If possible involve a friend or your spouse in your exercise program. Exercising with another person or a group can help you stay engaged. Research has found that adherence to an exercise program is much better when the exercise is performed with a friend or in a group. Plan to change your exercise routine about every six weeks. Keep it fresh and try new activities. If you can afford a personal trainer, this can be very helpful. A good personal trainer can set up a program that will meet your goals while keeping the exercise fun and interesting.

What Is the Best Time of Day to Exercise?

There are times when the body is more responsive to exercise than others. Not surprising this is due to the body's circadian rhythm. As you have seen, all physiological, neurological, and metabolic processes are controlled by the body's circadian rhythm. For example, resting metabolism and body temperature are highest in mid-afternoon and lowest in the early morning hours. Likewise, most cognitive functions peak in the late afternoon and early evening hours. The majority of physiological and metabolic rhythms associated with physical performance peak between 1:00 P.M. and 9:00 P.M. Strength, for example, peaks between 2:00 P.M. and 6:00 P.M. as does cardiovascular performance.

The relationship between time of day and gains in both aerobic capacity and strength has been well documented. Most people will find that exercising in the late afternoon places less stress on their body. The studies suggest that exercising when body temperature is at its highest may increase muscle flexibility, thereby reducing injuries and lessening postexercise muscle soreness.

When all is said and done, however, the best time to exercise is when you can schedule it. There are those early risers who find that exercising is the best way to get their day started. People who exercise in the morning tend to be more faithful to their exercise program. Determine whether you are a morning or afternoon exerciser, and then plan your exercise to accommodate your biorhythms if possible. If your schedule does not allow you to exercise according to your biorhythms, this is okay. The benefits of exercise are still the same. The main thing is to schedule your exercise program into each week and stick to it.

How Much Time Should I Exercise?

We recommend initially that you exercise for 30 minutes at a moderate level three to four times a week. This is equivalent to a brisk walk or jog of 2 to 2.5 miles. As you become better trained, increase your exercise duration and intensity for a more beneficial workout.

How Hard Should I Exercise?

When first getting started, select an exercise you feel comfortable doing and begin at an exercise intensity that allows you to exercise for 30 minutes without undue fatigue. As you become more conditioned, increase the intensity and duration of your exercising. Don't overdo it. Time is on your side.

Where Is the Best Place to Exercise?

Developing an exercise routine at home is a convenient option. Jogging, walking, and cycling are easy to do from home. You may also find it enjoyable to mix in some calisthenics such as push-ups, jumping jacks, deep-knee bends, pull-ups, toe raises, and some stretching exercises. There are many good exercise programs on DVD that can be purchased. For some ideas, see the Resources section on page 201. Most have progressive programs, which allow you to start slow and gradually increase the intensity of your workouts.

Joining a gym or health club is another option. The health club scene can be intimidating at first. You may not know how to use the equipment or may not be familiar with health club etiquette. What you need to realize is that most gym members were in your shoes when they first started. You will find that members are very willing to offer help if you ask. Furthermore, the employees are there to assist you and the well-run gyms or conditioning centers even provide courses to help new members get started. These programs include proper use of the equipment and development of an initial exercise program based on your personal goals.

We would recommend you visit three or four health clubs and talk with the managers. Find out what benefits are provided new members, and check out the equipment and the types of classes that are offered. Most health clubs have both resistance and aerobic exercise equipment, and the large conditioning centers also have pools and sport courts. Many of the larger centers also provide childcare.

What Is the Best Type of Exercise (Aerobic, Resistance, or Circuit Training)?

There are three basic exercise training programs: aerobic, resistance, and circuit training. Each one has specific advantages and limitations, which are discussed next and should be considered when developing your own program. Remember, the best exercise is the one that you will stay with. There are hundreds of ways you can incorporate exercise into your weekly routine. If you select one you enjoy, you'll stay committed and that is far more important than focusing on every muscle group. In the Hardwired Tool Kit, we've also outlined guidelines and exercises for aerobic-, resistance-, and circuit-training routines.

Aerobic Training

An aerobic training program exercises the cardiovascular system. Aerobic training strengthens the heart, reduces the buildup of fat deposits in the coronary arteries, lowers blood pressure, and improves muscle endurance. The heart is the most important muscle in the body. Without a strong heart, it does not matter if the other muscles of the body are fit. That's why all exercise programs should include an aerobic component.

Aerobic training is characterized by prolonged continuous exercise using large muscle groups. Examples of aerobic exercise are bicycling, jogging or running on a treadmill, using an elliptical trainer, cycling on a stationary bike, and swimming. Of course, aerobic exercise does not have to be performed in a gym. However, the advantages are that it is a safe environment, and the aerobic equipment generally provides excellent feedback on your performance during your workout by monitoring your heart rate, speed, and calories burned to name a few. Also, most aerobic equipment can be programmed so that you can gradually increase the difficulty of your exercise program progressively as your fitness level increases.

Resistance Training

Resistance training, also referred to as strength training, refers to movement against a resistance such as a weight or rubber band. The most popular type of resistance exercise is weightlifting. This can be done with free weights and/or weight machines. The benefits of resistance exercise are not the same as those for aerobic exercise, but they are just as important. Resistance exercise helps build muscle and develop strength; it increases bone density and strengthens connective tissue. These benefits are very important because around the age of 50 we start to lose muscle mass and strength, connective tissue becomes weaker and less flexible, and bone density declines. Resistance training can slow this aging process. Improvements in muscle strength also translate into better performance of everyday activities, such as climbing stairs, lifting children, and carrying bags of groceries. Stronger muscles also mean better mobility and balance, and thus a lower risk of falling and injuring yourself. More lean body mass aids in weight control because a pound of muscle burns substantially more calories than a pound of fat. Some researchers have even found that resistance exercise is more effective than aerobic exercise for weight loss.

Circuit Training

Circuit training combines aerobic and resistance exercises in one workout. For example, a circuit could consist of push-ups, sit-ups, pull-ups, lunges, rope jumping, shoulder presses, and rows. The benefits of circuit training exercise are that it burns a lot of calories in a short period of time, keeps the heart rate elevated, and develops muscle strength and tone. With circuit training, the idea is to complete one type of exercise right after the other with little or no rest in between. You try to do each exercise for a specified number of repetitions or within a specified time, and then move on to the next exercise. Completing all exercises is considered one circuit. Multiple circuits can be performed to increase exercise intensity and duration. A good circuit training program works all the major muscle groups, strengthens the cardiovascular system, and best yet gives you a quality workout in just 30 minutes.

EXTENDING THE BENEFITS OF EXERCISE

Regardless of the type of exercise you select, you can significantly boost its benefits by taking advantage of the postexercise metabolic window. In the 30 to 45 minutes after exercise, the circuits responsible for building muscle protein and replenishing muscle energy stores are activated. In fact, this period should be viewed as a fifth functional interval. Unlike the other functional intervals, which are defined by the body's circadian rhythm, the postexercise functional interval is determined by the time of the day you exercise. Like the other functional intervals, the postexercise interval offers you an opportunity to raise the efficiency of your fitness circuitry. Consuming the right combination of nutrients during this 30- to 45-minute window can increase lean body mass, reduce muscle soreness, and enable you to exercise the next time with more energy.

Drinking a carbohydrate-rich beverage, such as a sports drink, immediately after exercise can help you maximize these benefits. However, studies show that drinking a carbohydrate-rich beverage that contains a small amount of protein works much better. Ideally, the beverage or food consumed in the postexercise window should contain 70 to 80 percent carbohydrate and 20 to 30 percent protein, and should be about 100 to 120 calories. This small amount of postexercise nutrition will actually improve your body composition and accelerate your fitness development.

Whether your postexercise nutrition is a sports recovery drink, a recovery bar, or a combination of natural foods is unimportant. Beverages are more easily digested and also help to replenish fluids lost from sweating.

Finally, keep in mind that the postexercise window only stays open for 30 to 45 minutes. If you do not consume your nutrient-rich beverage during this time, you will miss all the metabolic benefits.

3. REDUCING YOUR DAILY CALORIC INTAKE

Small reductions in your daily caloric intake over the long-term produce more permanent changes in weight and improvements in body composition. In week five, you will reduce your daily caloric intake by 100 calories. In week six, you will make a second 100-calorie per day reduction. These small reductions do nut disrupt the normal functioning of your fitness circuits. As you saw in Chapter 1, when people attempt to lose weight by dramatically dropping their caloric intake by 700 to 1,200 calories a day, the body rebels. After the diet ends, they not only often gain more weight than they lost but they will have also lost valuable lean body mass.

A small reduction in calories, especially if gradually implemented, does not produce this compensatory response. A small reduction in calorie intake, especially after your circuits have been resynchronized, will scarcely be felt because you will have already gained the benefits of Functional Eating.

REVIEW YOUR FUNCTIONAL EATING PLAN

The best way to make this modest reduction in daily calories is to review your Functional Eating Plan. You can affect this change by reducing portion size or by simply dropping a food choice. You will go through the same process in week six. Both of these adjustments seem so minor that you are probably asking, "Is it worth the effort?" The answer is emphatically yes. This is part of switching your body into fitness mode. Also, whenever possible, try to include more and more super-functional foods in your daily diet; these foods have a heightened impact on your fitness circuitry.

SUMMARY

The main goals of Phase Two are to help you switch your body into fitness mode. This phase takes four weeks and involves making a few subtle changes in your daily activity and food choices. In weeks three and four, you focus on increasing your daily energy expenditure through a combination of lifestyle activity adjustments and the addition of an exercise regimen three to four times a week. In weeks five and six, you decrease your caloric intake by 100 calories each week. Each one of these changes independently improves the efficiency of your fitness circuits, but when you make all three the results can be dramatic not only in terms of fitness but also in terms of your overall health, quality of life, and longevity.

After four weeks in Phase Two, you are now on the fast track to fitness. The reason this program is vastly different from others you have tried is that now you have fine-tuned your body so that it is working with you to achieve your fitness goals (Figure 9.1). In other words, you are rolling that giant boulder downhill.

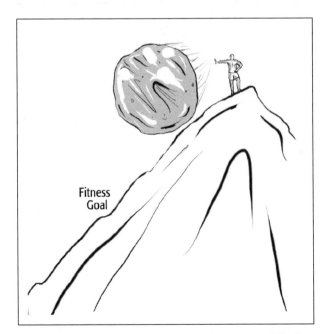

Figure 9.1. The result of working with your body's natural rhythm.

One cautionary note: It probably took you years to get into your current state of unfitness. You are not going to reverse this process in just a few weeks. We have cited many studies showing how fast the fitness circuits can become out of sync and how quickly one's fitness level can deteriorate. However, the reverse holds true. Once you resynchronize your circuits and switch your body into fitness mode, you will be amazed at the how fast your fitness level will improve. In Phase Three, you will really begin to notice changes as you continue to implement the program and monitor your progress. You shouldn't view the Hardwired Fitness Program as a six months' effort. You are now living a fitness lifestyle.

PHASE TWO: Switch Your Body into Fitness Mode

Week	Activities
Week 3	Raise threshold activity level by 100 calories per day.
Week 4	Add 30 minutes of moderate exercise 3 to 4 times a week.
Week 5	Decrease daily calorie intake by 100 calories per day.
Week 6	Decrease daily calorie intake by an additional 100 calories per day.

CHAPTER 10

Phase Three:
Get into the Red Zone

A popular descriptor often used in football is the "red zone." The red zone is defined as the area between the 20-yard line and the goal. When a team gets within an opponent's 20-yard line it has an excellent opportunity to score. The red zone is also a useful term to describe Phase Three of the Hardwired Fitness Program. In Phase One, you restored your body's natural balance. In Phase Two, you switched your body into fitness mode. To continue the football analogy, you have marched 80 yards down the field. You are in the red zone. Now it's time to defeat your opponent, who, in this case, is an unfit you. In Phase Three, you are going to see results; therefore, it's important to have a mechanism to assess your progress.

In the past, weight loss was your probable benchmark. It's an easy number to monitor; all you need is a scale. By now you realize that weight, although an important component of fitness, is just one of three key elements—body composition and activity capacity are the other two. We've created as assessment protocol so you can easily calculate your Hardwired Fitness Score. At weeks 7, 16, and 24, you will repeat the measurements. This will give you the positive incentive to stick with the program and encourage you to make additional modifications to help you get fit even faster. You will be amazed at how quickly you see results.

The two key steps of Phase Three are:

1. Calculate your baseline Hardwired Fitness Score.

2. Follow the program for an additional 17 weeks.

1. CALCULATING YOUR HARDWIRED FITNESS SCORE

Your Hardwired Fitness Score (HFS) is a composite of your BMI, percentage of body fat, and activity capacity (Figure 10.1). Each of these parameters can be assessed in an exercise physiology laboratory but that is both time-consuming and expensive. We have developed a simple but accurate alternative to enable you to calculate your HFS. The only tools you need are:

- A scale
- A tape measure
- A watch with a second hand
- A calculator

In this section we will walk you through how to calculate your HFS. The first time it may seem a little tedious since you have to make a number of calculations; the next assessment will be much easier. Record all your values on the HFS worksheet found on page 199 in the Hardwired Tool Kit.

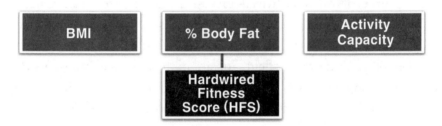

Figure 10.1. The Three Components of Your Hardwired Fitness Score.

DETERMINE YOUR BMI

BMI, even though it has limitations for people who are extremely tall, extremely muscular, or elderly, is an accurate reflection of the weight you should carry according to your height. To determine your BMI:

1. Weigh yourself on a scale.

2. Then, using the table in Figure 10.2, find your height (in inches) in the left-hand column. Move across to your weight (in pounds) and follow the column up. The number at the top is your BMI. For example, if you are 5 feet 4 inches (64 inches) tall and weigh 150 pounds, your BMI is 26.

As shown in Table 10.1, a BMI of 26 would put you in the overweight category.

Don't be discouraged if your BMI is much higher than you want. That's one of the reasons you are on this program. Record your BMI on the HFS worksheet.

Table 10.1. BMI Ranges

Weight Level	BMI Range	Weight Level	BMI Range
Underweight	Less than 18.5	Obese	30.0–35.0
Normal Weight	18.5–24.9	Morbidly Obese	Greater than 35.0
Overweight	25.0–29.9		

CALCULATE YOUR PERCENTAGE OF BODY FAT

The most accurate way to measure your percentage of body fat is by immersing yourself in water and measuring the amount of water you displace. Here is simpler but highly accurate method to determine your body fat percent:

1. Weigh yourself.

2. Measure your waist at the navel and record it in inches.

3. Using the calculator, plug the two values into the following formula:

For women:
   $[(4.15 \times \text{waist measurement}) - (0.082 \times \text{weight}) - 76.76] \div \text{weight}$

For men:
   $[(4.15 \times \text{waist measurement}) - (0.082 \times \text{weight}) - 98.42] \div \text{weight}$

The result is your percent of body fat. Record your percentage on the HFS worksheet.

Here is an example of the body-fat calculation for a 150-pound woman who has a 32-inch waist:

Body Mass Index Table

Height (inches)	BMI	Normal						Overweight					Obese										Extreme Obesity															
	BMI	19	20	21	22	23	24	25	26	27	28	29	30	31	32	33	34	35	36	37	38	39	40	41	42	43	44	45	46	47	48	49	50	51	52	53	54
													Body Weight (pounds)																								
58		91	96	100	105	110	115	119	124	129	134	138	143	148	153	158	162	167	172	177	181	186	191	196	201	205	210	215	220	224	229	234	239	244	248	253	258
59		94	99	104	109	114	119	124	128	133	138	143	148	153	158	163	168	173	178	183	188	193	198	203	208	212	217	222	227	232	237	242	247	252	257	262	267
60		97	102	107	112	118	123	128	133	138	143	148	153	158	163	168	174	179	184	189	194	199	204	209	215	220	225	230	235	240	245	250	255	261	266	271	276
61		100	106	111	116	122	127	132	137	143	148	153	158	164	169	174	180	185	190	195	201	206	211	217	222	227	232	238	243	248	254	259	264	269	275	280	285
62		104	109	115	120	126	131	136	142	147	153	158	164	169	175	180	186	191	196	202	207	213	218	224	229	235	240	246	251	256	262	267	273	278	284	289	295
63		107	113	118	124	130	135	141	146	152	158	163	169	175	180	186	191	197	203	208	214	220	225	231	237	242	248	254	259	265	270	278	282	287	293	299	304
64		110	116	122	128	134	140	145	151	157	163	169	174	180	186	192	197	204	209	215	221	227	232	238	244	250	256	262	267	273	279	285	291	296	302	308	314
65		114	120	126	132	138	144	150	156	162	168	174	180	186	192	198	204	210	216	222	228	234	240	246	252	258	264	270	276	282	288	294	300	306	312	318	324
66		118	124	130	136	142	148	155	161	167	173	179	186	192	198	204	210	216	223	229	235	241	247	253	260	266	272	278	284	291	297	303	309	315	322	328	334
67		121	127	134	140	146	153	159	166	172	178	185	191	198	204	211	217	223	230	236	242	249	255	261	268	274	280	287	293	299	306	312	319	325	331	338	344
68		125	131	138	144	151	158	164	171	177	184	190	197	203	210	216	223	230	236	243	249	256	262	269	276	282	289	295	302	308	315	322	328	335	341	348	354
69		128	135	142	149	155	162	169	176	182	189	196	203	209	216	223	230	236	243	250	257	263	270	277	284	291	297	304	311	318	324	331	338	345	351	358	365
70		132	139	146	153	160	167	174	181	188	195	202	209	216	222	229	236	243	250	257	264	271	278	285	292	299	306	313	320	327	334	341	348	355	362	369	376
71		136	143	150	157	165	172	179	186	193	200	208	215	222	229	236	243	250	257	265	272	279	286	293	301	308	315	322	329	338	343	351	358	365	372	379	386
72		140	147	154	162	169	177	184	191	199	206	213	221	228	235	242	250	258	265	272	279	287	294	302	309	316	324	331	338	346	353	361	368	375	383	390	397
73		144	151	159	166	174	182	189	197	204	212	219	227	235	242	250	257	265	272	280	288	295	302	310	318	325	333	340	348	355	363	371	378	386	393	401	408
74		148	155	163	171	179	186	194	202	210	218	225	233	241	249	256	264	272	280	287	295	303	311	319	326	334	342	350	358	365	373	381	389	396	404	412	420
75		152	160	168	176	184	192	200	208	216	224	232	240	248	256	264	272	279	287	295	303	311	319	327	335	343	351	359	367	375	383	391	399	407	415	423	431
76		156	164	172	180	189	197	205	213	221	230	238	246	254	263	271	279	287	295	304	312	320	328	336	344	353	361	369	377	385	394	402	410	418	426	435	443

Source: Adapted from Clinical Guidelines on the Identification, Evaluation, and Treatment of Overweight and Obesity in Adults: The Evidence Report.

Figure 10.2. Body Mass Index table.

$$[(4.15 \times 32) - (0.082 \times 150) - 76.76] \div 150$$
$$[132.8 - 12.30 - 76.76] \qquad \div 150$$
$$43.74 \qquad\qquad \div 150 = .29 \text{ or } 29\% \text{ body fat}$$

With a body-fat result of 29 percent, our female example would be at the high end of the normal range, as shown in Table 10.2.

Table 10.2. Percentage of Body Fat Classifications by Gender

Classification	Women (% Fat)	Men (% Fat)
Athletes	14–20%	6–13%
Fit Individuals	21–24%	14–17%
Normal Range	25–31%	18–25%

CALCULATE YOUR ACTIVITY CAPACITY

The final measurement in calculating your HFS is your activity capacity. Having good activity capacity enables you to perform your daily functions without fatigue. It enables you to respond appropriately when higher energy expenditure is required. A higher activity capacity enables you to enjoy more of life. A high-activity capacity also lowers the risk of many diseases, such as type 2 diabetes and coronary heart disease, and enables you to live longer.

For an elite athlete, activity capacity (also called aerobic capacity) is measured under carefully controlled conditions. The athlete either runs on a treadmill or pedals on a stationary bike at increasing levels of intensity. During the test, oxygen (carbon dioxide) and heart rate are measured. From these measurements activity capacity can be calculated.

Fortunately, there is a do-it-yourself test that allows you to measure your activity capacity. It is called the Rockport Test. Here's how you do it:

1. Walk a measured mile. It can be on a track, or along relatively flat ground or street.

2. Time how long it takes you to walk the measured mile. Convert the time into minutes using Table 10.3. For example, if your time is 17 minutes

20 seconds, you would use the table to convert 20 seconds into approximately 0.3 minutes. Your mile time would be recorded as 17.3 minutes. Jot down your converted time.

Table 10.3			
Seconds	Tenth of Minute	Seconds	Tenth of Minute
0–5	0.1	31–35	0.6
6–10	0.2	36–40	0.7
11–15	0.3	41–45	0.8
12–20	0.3	46–50	0.8
21–25	0.4	51–55	0.9
26–30	0.5	56–60	1.0

3. Immediately after the walk, record your heart rate. To do this, take a 15-second pulse count and multiply by 4 to calculate the beats per minute. Note: To count your pulse, stand quietly and place the tips of your first two fingers of one hand on the bottom side of the opposite wrist just below the thumb. You should feel a strong pulse. Count the pulse beats for 15 seconds. Jot down your heart rate.

4. To calculate your activity capacity, enter the information:

Age: _____ years

Weight: _____ lbs

Walk time: _____ minutes

Heart rate at the end of one mile: _____ beats per minute

Using the calculator, enter each value below and complete the calculation:

A = .077 × (body weight) _____ = _____

B = .39 × (age) _____ = _____

C = 3.26 × (1 mile walk time) _____ = _____

D = .16 × (1 minute heart rate) _____ = _____

Once you have calculated values for A, B, C and D, insert them into the following formula to determine your activity capacity:

- For women: Activity capacity = 132.85 − A − B − C − D
- For men: Activity capacity = 132.85 − A − B − C − D + 6.15

Compare your activity capacity value to the values in Table 10.4. A man age 35 with an activity capacity of 40.4 would be considered to have moderate activity capacity. For determining your Hardwired Fitness Score, we use your net activity capacity, which simply is 80 minus your activity capacity. For the example given above, the 35-year-old man would have a net activity capacity of 39.6 (80–40.4). Compute your net activity capacity and record the value on the HFS worksheet.

Table 10.4. Normal Activity Capacities by Age and Gender

		Women	Men
	Low Activity Capacity	< 30.6	< 37.1
Ages 20–29	Moderate Activity Capacity	30.6–36.6	37.1–44.2
	High Activity Capacity	36.7+	44.3+
	Low Activity Capacity	< 28.7	< 35.3
Ages 30–39	Moderate Activity Capacity	28.7–34.6	35.3–42.4
	High Activity Capacity	34.7+	42.5+
	Low Activity Capacity	< 26.5	< 33.0
Ages 40–49	Moderate Activity Capacity	26.5–32.3	33.0–39.9
	High Activity Capacity	32.4+	40.0+
	Low Activity Capacity	< 25.1	< 31.4
Ages 50–59	Moderate Activity Capacity	25.1–31.3	31.4–39.3
	High Activity Capacity	31.4+	39.4+
	Low Activity Capacity	< 21.9	< 28.3
Ages 60+	Moderate Activity Capacity	21.9–28.2	28.3–36.1
	High Activity Capacity	28.3+	36.2+

DETERMINE YOUR HARDWIRED FITNESS SCORE (HFS)

Your HFS is an accurate assessment of your fitness level. To arrive at your HFS, add your BMI, body fat percentage, and net activity capacity. Your HFS is a function of both your age and your gender. Once you have your HFS, refer to Table 10.5 (women) or 10.6 (men) for your fitness level. The lower your HFS, the greater your fitness level. The inset on page 163 describes how Mary G. determined her Hardwired Fitness Score.

Table 10.5. Hardwired Fitness Score (HFS)
FOR WOMEN

	Low Fit	Fit Range			High Fit
Age	Greater than	Moderately Low	Moderate	Moderately High	Less than
20–29	98	98–93	92–87	86–83	83
30–39	100	100–95	94–89	89–85	85
40–49	103	103–98	97–92	91–87	87
50–59	104	104–99	98–93	92–88	88
60+	107	107–102	101–96	95–91	91

Table 10.6. Hardwired Fitness Score (HFS)
FOR MEN

	Low Fit	Fit Range			High Fit
Age	Greater than	Moderately Low	Moderate	Moderately High	Less than
20–29	85	85–80	79–74	73–68	68
30–39	87	87–82	81–76	75–70	70
40–49	89	89–84	83–78	77–73	73
50–59	91	91–86	85–80	79–73	73
60+	94	94–89	88–84	83–76	76

Mary G. Determines
Her Hardwired Fitness Score

Mary G. is a 50-year-old woman who weighs 150 pounds. After walking a measured mile, she recorded her time in tenths of a minute. She also measured her pulse rate immediately after completing the mile. She recorded her results below:

Weight: 150

Age: 50

Walk time: 15 minutes 15 seconds = 15.3 minutes

Heart rate at the end of one mile: 125 beats per minute

Mary then computed the values below.

A = .077 × 150 (weight) = 11.5

B = .39 × 50 (age) = 19.5

C = 3.26 × 15.3 (walk time) = 49.8

D = .16 × 125 (beats per minute) = 20.6

Next she computed her activity capacity using the following formula for women:

132.8 − A − B − C − D

or

132.85 − 11.5(A) − 19.5(B) − 49.8(C) − 20.6(D) = 31.2

Based on Table 10.5, Mary G. with an activity capacity of 31.29 would have a moderate activity capacity. Her net activity capacity is 47.71 (80 − 31.29). The values for Mary G. HFS were:

BMI: 26

Fat %: 29

Net activity capacity: 47.7

HFS = 102.7

According to Table 10.5, Mary's HFS of 102.7 would be in the moderately low range of fitness.

2. THE HARDWIRED FITNESS 24-WEEK SCHEDULE

This section provides a detailed week-by-week activity list for all three phases. Most individuals start a fitness or weight-loss plan with great enthusiasm. Commitment to any program, no matter what it is, is usually very high at first—then enthusiasm wanes. Because the Hardwired Fitness Plan does not require dramatic changes to your lifestyle, it will be much easier to stick with it. It is probably also worthwhile to review the resolutions for success found in Chapter 7. As you start to see improvements in your daily energy level and body composition and weight, you will be continually remotivated to stay the course. Your confidence will build with each passing day. You will have made a painless but significant lifestyle change.

PHASE 1: RESTORE YOUR NATURAL METABOLIC RHYTHM

Week 1

1. Calculate your threshold level of activity.

2. Complete a Personal Energy Inventory.

3. If you are below your threshold level, modify your daily lifestyle by substituting net-positive for net-zero activities so that you reach your threshold level.

4. Make adjustments in your daily schedule to ensure you reach your threshold level of sleep.

Week 2

1. Determine your daily caloric needs.

2. Institute a functional meal plan based on your daily caloric needs. Pay particular attention to timing your meals to your body's natural functional rhythm.

PHASE 2: SWITCH YOUR BODY INTO FITNESS MODE

Week 3

1. Reevaluate your Personal Energy Inventory and make appropriate changes to increase your daily lifestyle activity by 100 calories per day.

Week 4

1. Start your exercise program consisting of 30 minutes of moderate exercise three to four times per week. After exercising, consume a carbohydrate/protein beverage or food as part of your routine.

Week 5

1. Review your Functional Meal Plan and make an appropriate change to reduce your caloric intake by 100 calories per day.

Week 6

1. Re-review your Functional Meal Plan and make a second reduction in your caloric intake of 100 calories per day.

PHASE 3: GET INTO THE RED ZONE

Week 7

1. Calculate your baseline Hardwired Fitness Score using the steps detailed in this chapter. Record your results on the HFS worksheet provided.

Weeks 8–15

1. Follow the program.

Week 16

1. Calculate your Hardwired Fitness Score to evaluate your progress. Record your results on the HFS worksheet provided.

Weeks 17–23

1. Follow the program.

Week 24

1. At the end of week 24, calculate your Hardwired Fitness Score. Record your results on the HFS worksheet provided.

Weeks 25 Onward

1. Evaluate your progress.

2. Recalculate your daily caloric needs using the worksheet on page 176 since your weight is now less. Make appropriate modifications in your meal plan based on this new value.

3. Increase your exercise activity by 35 to 45 minutes per week.

4. Make any other adjustments in your diet that you feel are necessary.

WHAT RESULTS CAN I EXPECT?

When your fitness circuitry becomes disconnected and your body becomes out of sync with its natural metabolic rhythm, it is remarkable how fast you can lose fitness. Anyone who has ever broken a bone that required immobilization with a cast is intimately familiar with how rapidly she or he loses strength and muscle mass. Lack of movement can cause a 25 percent loss of muscle mass in two weeks. The reverse also is true. Once your body switches into a fitness mode, you will begin to see changes very quickly. This is not to suggest that in 24 weeks you will restore your fitness to the same level as when you were a teenager. Remember, it took years for you to arrive at your current level of unfitness. The point being that when you create the proper conditions through activity, healthy nutrition, and meal timing, positive changes come quickly.

Here are some reasonable changes that you can expect after the first 24 weeks on the Hardwired Fitness Program:

- Weight loss of 7 to 20 pounds
- Decrease in body fat of 3 to 5 percent
- Reduction in waist circumference by several inches
- Increase of 10 to 20 percent in your activity capacity

In addition, many risk factors such as elevated blood pressure and poor blood lipid profile improve. After 24 weeks, you'll want to increase your exercise routine by 35 to 45 minutes per week. This will bring about even faster and greater benefits because, as we said previously, exercise is the gift that keeps on giving.

SUMMARY

Phase Three is when you'll really start to see results as measured by an improvement in your overall fitness level. In this phase, you assess your progress by seeing improvements in your Hardwired Fitness Score at weeks 7, 16, and 24. Over 24 weeks you will be surprised at the remarkable progress you make in terms of weight loss, increase in lean body mass, and improvement in activity capacity. Best of all, this transformation in your fitness will have taken place naturally without a major change in your lifestyle or eating habits.

PHASE THREE: Get into the Red Zone	
Week	Activities
Weeks 7–24	• Calculate your baseline Hardwired Fitness Score at weeks 7, 16, and 24.
	• Follow the program and enjoy the transformation.

CHAPTER 11

Hardwired Fitness Tool Kit

This chapter is your tool kit to make it very easy for you to implement the Hardwired Fitness Program. The kit contains the following tools:

1. Threshold Activity Worksheet

2. Calorie Expenditure for Common Lifestyle and Occupational Activities.

3. Calculating Daily Caloric Needs

4. Hardwired Fitness Meal Plans
   - 1,800 calories per day
   - 2,000 calories per day
   - 2,300 calories per day
   - 2,500 calories per day
   - 2,800 calories per day
   - 3,000 calories per day

5. Super-Functional Foods

6. Combining Lifestyle Activity and Exercise

7. Exercise Programs
   - Aerobic
   - Cross Training
   - Resistance

8. Hardwired Fitness Score Worksheet

9. Resources

1. THRESHOLD ACTIVITY WORKSHEET

Determine Your Minimum Threshold Activity Level

1. Find your weight in the appropriate Table 11.1 below and multiply it by the constant in the right-hand column.

2. Record your Minimum Threshold Activity Level: _____

Table 11.1. Threshold Activity Level by Gender

Women		Men	
Weight	Multiplier	Weight	Multiplier
Below 120	5.4	Below 120	6.0
120–145	5.2	121–145	5.8
146–165	4.7	146–175	5.2
166–190	4.4	176–200	4.9
191–230	4.0	201–230	4.8
Above 230	3.8	Above 230	4.7

Conduct a Personal Energy Inventory

1. Record your current weight in column A in Table 11.2.

2. Using the listing on page 172, select the lifestyle and occupational activities that are closest to your own daily activities.

3. Write down the net calories expended for the activity you selected in column B. Do this for each activity for all the time you are awake each day. Record your activities in no less than 15-minute intervals.

4. Estimate the number of minutes you spend on each activity and write the value for each activity in column C.

5. For each activity, multiply your weight (column A), times the net calories expended (column B) times the minutes (column C). Record the value in the total calories expended column (D).

6. Total up your minutes. Assuming you sleep 8 hours/day this value should equal 960 minutes.

7. Total up all the calories expended for each activity (column D). This is your lifestyle calorie expenditure.

Table 11.2. Personal Energy Inventory

Activity	A. Weight (pounds)	B. Net Calories Expended	C. Time (minutes)	D. Total Calories Expended (A x B x C)
TOTAL				

Determine If You Reach Your Threshold Level

1. Compare your Minimum Threshold Activity Level computed in Part 1 of this worksheet with the Total Lifestyle Calorie Expenditure computed in Part 2. If your Total Lifestyle Calorie Expenditure exceeds your Minimum Threshold Activity Level that is excellent. You still might wish to analyze your Personal Energy Inventory to see how you might improve it.

2. If your Total Lifestyle Calorie Expenditure is less than your Minimum Threshold Activity Level, you must make appropriate modifications. Net-zero or low-calorie expenditure activities are the best place to start. See how you can substitute the time spent in these activities in whole or in part with higher calorie activities. Refer to the Calorie Expenditure for Common Lifestyle and Occupational Activities (Table 11.3) to help you.

3. After making appropriate modifications on your Personal Energy Inventory Worksheet recalculate your Total Lifestyle Calorie Expenditure to make sure you meet or exceed your Minimum Threshold Activity Level.

4. This is not a paper exercise. After creating your new Personal Energy Inventory make sure you are putting it into daily practice.

2. CALORIE EXPENDITURE FOR COMMON LIFESTYLE AND OCCUPATIONAL ACTIVITIES

Table 11.3 below lists many common lifestyle and occupational activities. You may not find activities specifically relevant to you. If so, select one that seems closest.

Table 11.3.

Activity	Net Calories Expended (cal/lb body weight/ minute activity)
Sleeping	0
Lying quietly, doing nothing, lying in bed awake, listening to music	0
Lying quietly, watching television	0
Meditating	0
Reclining and reading	0
Reclining and talking or talking on the phone	0
Reclining and writing	0
Riding in a car, bus, or truck	0
Sitting quietly and watching television	0
Sitting quietly, listening to music (not talking or reading), watching TV	0
Carpentry, general	0.019

Activity	Net Calories Expended (cal/lb body weight/ minute activity)
Standing quietly (standing in a line)	0.001
Sitting and reading, book, newspaper, etc.	0.002
Sitting and card playing, playing board games	0.004
Sitting and talking or talking on the phone	0.004
Sitting at a sporting event, spectator	0.004
Sitting at meetings, general, and/or with talking involved, eating at a business lunch	0.004
Typing computer	0.004
Watering lawn or garden, standing or walking	0.004
Sitting and studying, general, including reading and/or writing	0.006
Sitting and writing, desk work, typing	0.006
Sitting in class, general, including note taking or class discussion	0.006
Standing and talking or talking on the phone	0.006
Driving a car	0.007
Making bed	0.007
Sitting and doing arts and crafts, moderate effort	0.007
Standing during miscellaneous activities	0.007
Walking on job, less than 2.0 mph (in office or lab area), slowly	0.007
Walking, less than 2.0 mph, level ground, strolling, slowly	0.007
Cooking or food preparation and standing or sitting in general	0.007
Food shopping with or without a grocery cart, standing or walking	0.009
Non-food shopping, standing or walking	0.009
Standing; light (e.g., bartending, store clerk, assembling, filing, duplicating,	0.009
Cleaning, light (e.g., dusting, straightening up, changing linen, carrying out trash)	0.011
Custodial work, cleaning sink and toilet, light effort	0.011
Farming, driving tractor	0.011
Mowing lawn, riding mower	0.011
Multiple household tasks all at once, light effort	0.011
Operating heavy-duty equipment/automated, not driving	0.011
Putting away groceries (e.g., carrying groceries, shopping without a grocery cart)	0.011
Serving food, setting table (implied walking or standing)	0.011
Washing dishes; clearing dishes from table, walking	0.011
Sitting while playing with child(ren); light, only active periods	0.011

Activity	Net Calories Expended (cal/lb body weight/ minute activity)
Walk/run, playing with animals, light, only active periods	0.013
Walking, 2.5 mph, downhill	0.013
Child care: standing while dressing, bathing, grooming, feeding, occasional lifting	0.015
Cleaning, heavy or major (e.g., washing car, washing windows, cleaning garage), vigorous	0.015
Driving heavy truck, tractor, bus	0.015
Loading/unloading a car	0.015
Walking the dog	0.015
Walking, 2.5 mph, firm surface	0.015
Carpet sweeping, sweeping floors	0.017
Walking on job, 3.0 mph, in office, moderate speed, not carrying anything	0.017
Walking, 3.0 mph, level, moderate pace, firm surface	0.017
Carrying infant or 15-pound load (e.g., suitcase), level ground or downstairs	0.019
Electrical work, plumbing	0.019
Multiple household tasks all at once, moderate effort	0.019
Standing while packing/unpacking boxes, occasional lifting of household items	0.019
Trimming shrubs or trees, power cutter, using leaf blower, edger	0.019
Vacuuming	0.019
Scrubbing floors on hands and knees, scrubbing bathroom, bathtub	0.021
Walking on job, 3.5 mph, in office, brisk speed, not carrying anything	0.021
Walking, 3.5 mph, briskly, level firm surface, walking for exercise	0.021
Custodial work, feathering arena floor, moderate effort	0.022
Gardening, general	0.022
Lifting items continuously, 10–20 lbs, with limited walking or resting	0.022
Masseur, masseuse (standing)	0.022
Raking lawn	0.022
Sacking grass, leaves	0.022
Standing; moderate/heavy (e.g., lifting more than 50 lbs, masonry, painting, paper)	0.022
Walk/run, playing with animals, moderate, only active periods	0.022
Walking, 3.0 mph, moderately and carrying light objects less than 25 lbs	0.022
Standing; moderate/heavy (e.g., lifting more than 50 lbs, masonry, painting, paper)	0.022
Mowing lawn, power mower	0.026

Activity	Net Calories Expended (cal/lb body weight/ minute activity)
Carrying 1 to 15 lb load, upstairs	0.030
Carrying, loading, or stacking wood, loading/unloading or carrying lumber	0.030
Digging, spading, filling garden, composting	0.030
Forestry, ax chopping, slow	0.030
Using crutches	0.030
Walk/run while playing with child(ren), vigorous, only active periods	0.030
Walk/run, playing with animals, vigorous, only active periods	0.030
Walking or walk downstairs or standing, carrying objects about 25 to 49 lbs	0.030
Walking, 4.0 mph, level, firm surface, very brisk pace	0.030
Construction, outside, remodeling	0.034
Farming, shoveling grain, moderate effort	0.033
Mowing lawn, general	0.033
Chopping wood, splitting logs	0.037
Farming, taking care of animals (e.g., grooming, brushing, shearing sheep)	0.037
Forestry, planting by hand	0.037
Gardening with heavy power tools, tilling a garden, chain saw	0.037
Hiking, cross country	0.037
Moving furniture, household items, carrying boxes	0.037
Shoveling snow, by hand	0.037
Shoveling, light (less than 10 lbs/minute)	0.037
Using heavy power tools such as pneumatic tools (jackhammers, drills, etc.)	0.037
Walking, 3.5 mph, uphill	0.037
Hiking, cross country	0.037
Walking, 4.5 mph, level, firm surface, very, very brisk	0.040
Truck driving, loading and unloading truck (standing)	0.041
Walking or walking downstairs or standing, carrying objects about 50 to 74 lbs	0.041
Masonry or concrete work	0.045
Carrying groceries upstairs	0.048
Walking or walking downstairs or standing, carrying objects about 75 to 99 lbs	0.048
Walking, 5.0 mph	0.052
Walking upstairs	0.052
Operating snowblower	0.026
Walking, 3.5 mph, briskly and carrying objects less than 25 lbs	0.026

3. CALCULATING DAILY CALORIC NEEDS

Calculating your daily caloric needs is the first step in creating your Functional Eating Plan. To do this you must know your Daily Caloric Expenditure. This is the sum of your Minimum Threshold Activity Expenditure, plus your Resting Calorie Expenditure. This value will tell you what your calorie consumption should be to ensure that your body is in energy balance.

Table 11.4. Resting Caloric Expenditure

Women		Men	
Weight	Multiplier	Weight	Multiplier
Below 120	11.2	Below 120	12.2
120–130	10.5	120–135	11.7
131–150	9.8	136–160	10.9
151–175	9.1	161–185	10.3
176–210	8.4	186–210	9.8
214–230	7.8	211–230	9.3
Above 230	7.5	Above 230	9.0

Table 11.5. Minimum Threshold Activity Expenditure

Women		Men	
Weight	Multiplier	Weight	Multiplier
Below 120	5.5	Below 120	6.2
120–145	5.2	121–145	5.8
146–165	4.7	146–175	5.2
166–190	4.4	176–200	4.9
191–230	4.0	201–230	4.8
Above 230	3.8	Above 230	4.7

1. To compute your Resting Caloric Expenditure, use Table 11.4. Find

your weight in the appropriate section and multiply it by the value in the right-hand column.

2. To compute your Minimum Threshold Activity Expenditure, use Table 11.5. Find your weight in the appropriate section and multiply by the value in the right-hand column.

3. Add the two values to arrive at your Daily Caloric Needs.

Resting Caloric Expenditure: _____*1547*_____

+ Minimum Threshold Activity Expenditure: _____*748*_____

= Daily Caloric Needs _____*2295*_____

4. HARDWIRED FITNESS MEAL PLANS

The following Hardwired Fitness Meal Plans were created by Brittany Crim, a registered dietician who has extensive experience in weight management and fitness nutrition. She is currently at the University of Texas in Austin in the Department of Kinesiology and Health Education.

Brittany has developed meal plan options for a wide range of calorie levels: 1,800, 2,000, 2,300, 2,500, 2,800, and 3,000. They are intended to give you ideas for healthful meals. You can substitute any food as long as the substituted food is consistent with the recommended calories and macronutrient percent. There are many excellent websites that can help you plan meals that are consistent with the core principles of Functional Eating. You can find this information in the Resources section of the tool kit on page 201.

MASHED POTATOES
Yield: Two ½-cup servings

1 cup boiled potatoes
⅛ cup skim milk
1 tablespoon butter
Salt and freshly ground
  pepper to taste

½ cup = 110 kcal

CREAMED SPINACH
Yield: Two 1-cup servings

⅖ cup whole milk
1 10-ounce box frozen
  chopped spinach,
  thawed and squeezed
  dry (reserve ⅛-cup
  liquid)
½ large garlic cloves,
  minced
1 teaspoon butter

2 teaspoons all-purpose
  flour
⅛ cup grated
  Parmesan cheese
⅛ teaspoon ground
  nutmeg
Salt and freshly ground
  pepper to taste

1 cup = 130 kcal

1,800-CALORIES-PER-DAY MEAL PLAN OPTIONS
INTERVAL

	RESTORATION 7:00–9:00 a.m.	ACTIVITY Noon–2:00 p.m.
Calories: **Carbohydrate:** **Protein:** **Fat:**	368 60% 20% 20%	595 62% 7% 31%
Option 1	2 cups Cheerios or a comparable cereal 12 ounces 1% milk	$^2/_3$ cup hummus 1 6-inch whole-wheat pita pocket Small salad consisting of: 　1 cup mixed salad greens 　1 tablespoon Italian dressing 　10 ounces pomegranate juice
Option 2	English muffin 1 tablespoon reduced-fat peanut butter $^1/_2$ cup fresh strawberries 8 ounces 1% milk	PB&J sandwich consisting of: 　2 slices of whole-wheat bread 　1 tablespoon peanut butter 　1 tablespoon grape jelly $^1/_2$ cup applesauce
Option 3	Breakfast taco consisting of: 　1 6-inch flour tortilla 　3 egg whites 　$^1/_2$ ounces cheddar cheese 　10 ounces orange juice	Spaghetti consisting of: 　1 cup cooked spaghetti 　$^1/_2$ cup spaghetti sauce 　5–7 spears steamed asparagus with 　2 teaspoons olive oil 　7 ounces grape juice
Option 4	Peanut butter toast consisting of: 　2 slices whole-wheat toast 　1 tablespoon peanut butter 　$^1/_4$ cup fat-free cottage cheese 　$^2/_3$ cup mandarin orange slices	Mixed rice consisting of: 　1 cup cooked brown rice with 　1 tablespoon butter 　$^1/_2$ cup cooked corn 　10 ounces orange juice
Option 5	$^3/_4$ cup low-fat yogurt $^3/_4$ cup blackberries 1 cup cooked oatmeal	Mixed rice consisting of: 　1 cup cooked brown rice with 　1 tablespoon butter 　$^1/_2$ cup cooked black beans 　8 ounces cranberry juice

1,800-CALORIES-PER-DAY MEAL PLAN OPTIONS
INTERVAL

ACTIVITY 3:00–5:00 p.m.	REBUILDING 5:00–8:00 p.m.	ANTI-STRESS 8:00–11:00 p.m.
100 51% 23% 26%	648 25% 35% 40%	100 20% 80% 0%
1 stick light string cheese $3/4$ cup cubed cantaloupe	6 ounces top sirloin steak (lean), grilled or broiled $1/2$ cup mashed potatoes* $3/4$ cup creamed spinach* Reduced-fat fudge bar	4 ounces roasted turkey breast
5 2-inch reduced-fat wheat crackers $1/2$ ounce low-fat cheddar cheese	Cheeseburger consisting of: 1 whole-wheat hamburger bun 5 ounces ground round beef 1 ounce mozzarella cheese Pickles, onions, lettuce, tomato 1 cup steamed broccoli with 1 teaspoon butter	$3/4$ cup fat-free cottage cheese
$1^1/2$ ounces roasted chicken breast 3 ounces orange juice	Spanish chicken consisting of: 7 ounces grilled chicken breast, seared with $3/4$ tablespoon olive oil $1/2$ cup diced tomatoes $1/2$ cup cooked black beans 1 ounce cheddar cheese $1/4$ cup crushed tortilla strips	2 scoops vanilla whey protein power Water
	7 ounces pork chop, grilled or baked, drizzled with $3/4$ tablespoon olive oil $3/4$ cup cooked brown rice with $1/2$ tablespoon butter $1/4$ cup chocolate ice cream	
	7 ounces salmon, grilled or baked, with 1 teaspoon butter 1 cup cooked wild rice 1 cup steamed broccoli	

* See page 177 for Mashed Potato and Creamed Spinach recipes

2,000-CALORIES-PER-DAY MEAL PLAN OPTIONS
INTERVAL

	RESTORATION 7:00–9:00 a.m.	ACTIVITY Noon–2:00 p.m.
Calories: Carbohydrate: Protein: Fat:	420 60% 20% 20%	680 62% 7% 31%
Option 1	$2^1/_2$ cups Cheerios or a comparable cereal 12 ounces 1% milk	2 slices whole-wheat bread Large salad consisting of: 3 cups chopped vegetables such as: $^1/_2$ cup tomatoes $^1/_2$ cup brussels sprouts $^1/_2$ cup spinach $^1/_4$ cup cucumber 1 tablespoon olive $1^1/_4$ cups baby carrots with 1 tablespoon ranch dressing 2 cups diced fresh fruit 8 ounces grapefruit juice
Option 2	English muffin 1 teaspoon butter 2 slices Canadian bacon, grilled	PB&J sandwich consisting of: 2 slices of whole-wheat bread $2^1/_2$ tablespoons peanut butter 1 tablespoon grape jelly 16 ounces apple juice
Option 3	Breakfast taco consisting of: 1 6-inch flour tortilla 3 egg whites 1 ounce cheddar cheese 12 ounces orange juice	$^2/_3$ cup hummus 1 6-inch whole-wheat pita pocket Small salad consisting of: 1 cup mixed salad greens $^1/_4$ cup diced avocado 1 tablespoon Italian dressing 10 ounces pomegranate juice
Option 4	Peanut butter toast consisting of: 2 slices whole-wheat toast $^1/_2$ tablespoon peanut butter $^1/_2$ cup 2% cottage cheese $1^1/_2$ cups mandarin orange slices	Spaghetti consisting of: 1 cup cooked spaghetti $^1/_2$ cup spaghetti sauce 5–7 spears asparagus grilled with 1 tablespoon olive oil 8 ounces grape juice
Option 5	2 cooked eggs, any style $^1/_2$ grapefruit $^1/_4$ cup low-fat granola 8 ounces apple juice	Vegetarian wraps consisting of: 2 6-inch flour tortilla $^1/_2$ avocado $^1/_4$ cup salsa Lettuce, tomatoes, onions, peppers 3 fruit-and-cake cookies 1 large apple

2,000-CALORIES-PER-DAY MEAL PLAN OPTIONS
INTERVAL

ACTIVITY 3:00–5:00 p.m.	REBUILDING 5:00–8:00 p.m.	ANTI-STRESS 8:00–11:00 p.m.
100 51% 23% 26%	740 25% 35% 40%	100 20% 80% 0%

1 stick light string cheese
3/4 cup cubed cantaloupe
	6 ounces top sirloin steak (lean),
	  grilled or broiled
	1/2 cup mashed potatoes*
	1 1/2 cups creamed spinach*
	Reduced-fat fudge bar
		4 ounces roasted
		  turkey breast

5 2-inch reduced-fat wheat crackers
1/2 ounce low-fat cheddar cheese
	Cheeseburger consisting of:
	  1 whole-wheat hamburger bun
	  5 ounces ground round beef
	  1 ounce mozzarella cheese
	  Pickles, onions, lettuce, tomato
	1 1/2 cups steamed broccoli
	2 teaspoons butter
		3/4 cup fat-free
		  cottage cheese

1 1/2 ounces roasted chicken breast
3 ounces orange juice
	Spanish chicken consisting of:
	  7 ounces grilled chicken breast,
	  seared with 1 tablespoon olive oil
	1/2 cup diced tomatoes
	3/4 cup cooked black beans
	1 ounce cheddar cheese
	1/4 cup crushed tortilla strips
		2 scoops vanilla
		  whey protein
		  power
		Water

	7 ounces pork chop, baked with
	  3/4 tablespoon olive oil
	3/4 cup cooked brown rice with
	  1/2 tablespoon butter
	1 cup broccoli with 1 teaspoon butter	

	7 ounces salmon, grilled or baked with 1 teaspoon butter 1 1/2 cup cooked wild rice 1 cup steamed broccoli	

* See page 177 for Mashed Potato and Creamed Spinach recipes

2,300-CALORIES-PER-DAY MEAL PLAN OPTIONS
INTERVAL

	RESTORATION 7:00–9:00 a.m.	ACTIVITY Noon–2:00 p.m.
Calories: Carbohydrate: Protein: Fat:	473 60% 20% 20%	765 62% 7% 31%

Option 1	2 cups Cheerios or a comparable cereal
	12 ounces 1% milk
	6 ounces low-fat yogurt
		$^2/_3$ cup hummus
		1 whole-wheat pita pocket
		Small salad consisting of:
		   2 cups mixed salad greens
		   $^1/_2$ cup diced avocado
		   1 tablespoon Italian dressing
		14 ounces pomegranate juice

Option 2	Breakfast sandwich consisting of:
	  English muffin
	  1 teaspoon butter
	  2 slices grilled Canadian bacon
	  8 ounces skim milk
	  $1^1/_2$ cups blackberries
		PB&J sandwich consisting of:
		  2 slices of whole-wheat bread
		  3 tablespoons peanut butter
		  2 tablespoons grape jelly
		  16 ounces apple juice

Option 3	Breakfast taco consisting of:
	  1 6-inch flour tortilla
	  3 egg whites
	  1 ounce cheddar cheese
	  1 small plum
	  8 ounces grape juice
		Vegetarian tacos consisting of:
		  1 6-inch flour tortillas
		  $^3/_4$ cup cooked black beans
		  $^1/_3$ cup rice
		  1 cup green leaf lettuce
		  1 tablespoon butter (for tortillas and rice)
		  8 ounces cranberry juice

Option 4	Peanut butter toast consisting of:
	  2 slices whole-wheat toast
	  1 tablespoon peanut butter
	  $^1/_2$ cup 2% cottage cheese
	  $1^1/_2$ cups mandarin orange slices
		Spaghetti consisting of:
		  1 cup cooked spaghetti
		  $^1/_2$ cup spaghetti sauce
		  5–7 spears steamed asparagus with
		  1 tablespoon olive oil
		  4 ounces 1% milk
		  9 prunes

Option 5	2 eggs, cooked any style
	$^1/_2$ grapefruit
	$^1/_4$ cup low-fat granola
	$^3/_4$ cup fat-free, sugar-free yogurt
	8 ounces apple juice
		Vegetarian wraps consisting of:
		  2 6-inch flour tortilla
		  $^1/_2$ avocado
		  $^1/_4$ cup salsa
		  Lettuce, tomatoes, onions, peppers
		  3 fruit-and-cake cookies
		  1 large apple

2,300-CALORIES-PER-DAY MEAL PLAN OPTIONS
INTERVAL

ACTIVITY 3:00–5:00 p.m.	REBUILDING 5:00–8:00 p.m.	ANTI-STRESS 8:00–11:00 p.m.
100 51% 23% 26%	833 25% 35% 40%	100 20% 80% 0%
1 stick light string cheese $^3/_4$ cup cubed cantaloupe	8 ounces top sirloin steak (lean), grilled or broiled $^1/_2$ cup mashed potatoes* $^3/_4$ cup creamed spinach* $^1/_2$ ounce cheddar cheese 6 ounces apple juice	4 ounces roasted turkey breast

5 2-inch reduced-fat wheat crackers
$^1/_2$ ounce low-fat cheddar cheese
	Cheeseburger consisting of:
	  1 whole-wheat hamburger bun
	  7 ounces ground round beef
	  2 ounces mozzarella cheese
	  Pickles, onions, lettuce, tomato
	$^1/_2$ cup steamed broccoli with 1
	  teaspoon butter
	8 ounces 1% milk
		$^3/_4$ cup fat-free
		cottage cheese

1$^1/_2$ ounces roasted chicken breast 3 ounces orange juice	7 ounces braised pork rump roast $^1/_2$ cup cooked black beans $^1/_2$ cups steamed green beans	2 scoops vanilla whey protein power Water

	Spanish chicken consisting of:
	  7 ounces grilled chicken breast,
	  seared with 1 tablespoon olive oil
	  1 cup cooked black beans
	  1$^1/_2$ ounces cheddar cheese
	$^1/_2$ cup diced tomatoes
	$^1/_4$ cup crushed tortilla strips	

	Sandwich consisting of:
	  2 slices whole-wheat bread
	  7 ounces turkey breast
	  3 slices Genoa salami
	  1 ounce cheddar cheese
	  1 tablespoon mayonnaise
	  2 medium kiwi	

* See page 177 for Mashed Potato and Creamed Spinach recipes

2,500-CALORIES-PER-DAY MEAL PLAN OPTIONS
INTERVAL

	RESTORATION 7:00–9:00 a.m.	ACTIVITY Noon–2:00 p.m.
Calories: Carbohydrate: Protein: Fat:	525 60% 20% 20%	850 62% 7% 31%
Option 1	2 cups Cheerios or a comparable cereal 12 ounces 1% milk $1/_3$ cup plain, low-fat yogurt $1/_2$ cup strwberries	Large salad consisting of: 3 cups green leaf lettuce $1/_2$ cup cooked black beans $1/_2$ cup diced onions 1 cup sliced bell pepper 1 cup halved cherry tomatoes 2 tablespoons olive oil dressing with 1 tablespoon vinegar 1 slice whole-wheat bread 12 ounces grape juice
Option 2	1 cup cooked oatmeal with 1 teaspoon butter Peanut butter toast consisting of: 2 slices whole-wheat toast $1/_2$ tablespoon peanut butter $1/_2$ medium grapefruit $1/_2$ cup low-fat cottage cheese Coffee with $1/_2$ tablespoon fat-free French vanilla creamer	$2/_3$ cup hummus 1 whole-wheat pita pocket Small salad consisting of: 2 cups mixed salad greens $1/_2$ cup diced avocado 1 tablespoon Italian dressing 16 ounces pomegranate juice
Option 3	1 instant oatmeal packet with maple and brown sugar 1 slice of whole-wheat toast 1 large banana 2 whole large eggs and 2 large egg whites, scrambled	Stuffed baked potato consisting of: 1 large baked potato 1 cup steamed broccoli 1 tablespoon butter 2 tablespoons sour cream 1 medium peach 14-ounce vegetable and fruit fusion drink
Option 4	Breakfast taco consisting of: 1 6-inch flour tortilla 3 large egg whites 1 ounce turkey sausage $1/_2$ ounce cheddar cheese 8 ounces orange juice 1 large apple	Eggplant pasta consisting of: $1^1/_3$ cup cooked angel hair pasta 1 cup eggplant, sautéed with $1^1/_4$ tablespoon olive oil, plus Italian herbs and garlic to taste 12 ounces blackberries 8 ounces pineapple juice
Option 5	2 eggs, cooked any style $1/_2$ grapefruit $1/_4$ cup low-fat granola $3/_4$ cup fat-free, sugar-free yogurt 8 ounces apple juice	Vegetarian taco consisting of: 2 6-inch flour tortillas 1 tablespoon butter (for tortillas and rice) 1 cup cooked black beans $1/_3$ cup cooked brown rice 1 cup green leaf lettuce $1/_4$ cup diced avocado $1/_2$ cup mango salsa 8 ounces grapefruit juice

2,500-CALORIES-PER-DAY MEAL PLAN OPTIONS
INTERVAL

ACTIVITY 3:00–5:00 p.m.	REBUILDING 5:00–8:00 p.m.	ANTI-STRESS 8:00–11:00 p.m.
100 51% 23% 26%	925 25% 35% 40%	100 20% 80% 0%

1 stick light string cheese
³/₄ cup cubed cantaloupe
	8 ounces top sirloin steak (lean), grilled
	  or broiled
	¹/₂ cup mashed potatoes*
	³/₄ cup creamed spinach*
	1 ounce cheddar cheese
	1 ear corn on the cob
		4 ounces roasted
		  turkey breast

5 2-inch reduced-fat wheat crackers
¹/₂ ounce low-fat cheddar cheese
	Cheeseburger consisting of:
	  1 whole-wheat hamburger bun
	  7 ounces ground round beef
	  2 ounces mozzarella cheese
	  Pickles, onions, lettuce, tomato
	  ¹/₂ cup steamed broccoli with 1 teaspoon
	  butter
	  8 ounces 1% milk
		³/₄ cup fat-free
		  cottage cheese

1¹/₂ ounces roasted chicken breast
3 ounces orange juice
	8 ounces braised pork rump roast
	¹/₂ cup cooked black beans
	¹/₂ cups steamed green beans
	1- to 2-inch square of cornbread
		2 scoops vanilla
		  whey protein
		  power
		  Water

	Spanish chicken consisting of:
	  7 ounces grilled chicken breast, seared
	  with 1 tablespoon olive oil
	  1 cup cooked black beans
	  2 ounces cheddar cheese
	  ¹/₄ cup crushed tortilla strips	

	Sandwich consisting of:
	  2 slices whole-wheat bread
	  7 ounces turkey breast
	  2 slices Genoa salami
	  2 ounces cheddar cheese
	  1 tablespoon mayonnaise
	  2¹/₂ cups strawberries	

* See page 177 for Mashed Potato and Creamed Spinach recipes

2,800-CALORIES-PER-DAY MEAL PLAN OPTIONS
INTERVAL

	RESTORATION 7:00–9:00 a.m.	ACTIVITY Noon–2:00 p.m.
Calories: **Carbohydrate:** **Protein:** **Fat:**	578 60% 20% 20%	935 62% 7% 31%
Option 1	2 cups Cheerios or a comparable cereal 12 ounces 1% milk $^1/_3$ cup plain, low-fat yogurt 1 cup strawberries	Large salad consisting of: 3 cups green leaf lettuce $^1/_2$ cup cooked black beans $^1/_2$ cup corn $^1/_2$ cup diced onions 1 cup sliced bell pepper 1 cup halved cherry tomatoes 2 tablespoons olive oil dressing with 1 tablespoon vinegar 2 slices whole-wheat bread

Option 2	1 cup cooked oatmeal
	Peanut butter toast consisting of:
	  2 slices whole-wheat toast
	  1 tablespoon peanut butter
	$^1/_2$ medium grapefruit
	$^1/_2$ cup low-fat cottage cheese
	Coffee with $^1/_2$ tablespoon fat-free
	  French vanilla creamer
		$^2/_3$ cup hummus
		1 whole-wheat pita pocket
		Small salad consisting of:
		  2 cups mixed salad greens
		  $^1/_2$ cup diced avocado
		  1 tablespoon Italian dressing
		16 ounces pomegranate juice

Option 3	1 instant oatmeal packet with maple
	  and brown sugar
	1 slice of whole-wheat toast
	1 plum
	1 whole large egg with
	1 large egg whites, scrambled
	2 slices grilled Canadian bacon
		Stuffed baked potato consisting of:
		  1 large baked potato
		  1 cup steamed broccoli
		  1 tablespoon butter
		  2 tablespoons sour cream
		$^1/_2$ ounce honey-roasted cashews (about 9 nuts)
		1 medium peach
		16-ounce vegetable and fruit fusion drink

Option 4	2 eggs, cooked any style
	$^1/_2$ grapefruit
	$^1/_2$ cup low-fat granola
	$^3/_4$ cup fat-free, yogurt
	8 ounces apple juice
		Eggplant pasta consisting of:
		  1$^1/_3$ cup cooked angel hair pasta
		  1 cup eggplant, sautéed with 1$^1/_4$ tablespoon
		  olive oil, plus Italian herbs and garlic to taste
		1$^1/_2$ cups blackberries
		8 ounces pineapple juice
		$^1/_2$ ounce honey-roasted cashews (about 9 nuts)

Option 5	Breakfast taco consisting of:
	  1 6-inch flour tortilla
	  3 large egg whites
	  2 ounces turkey sausage
	  $^1/_4$ ounce cheddar cheese
	10 ounces orange juice
	1 large apple
		Vegetarian taco consisting of:
		  2 6-inch flour tortillas
		  1 tablespoon butter (for tortillas and rice)
		  1 cup cooked black beans
		  $^1/_3$ cup cooked brown rice
		  1 cup green leaf lettuce
		  $^1/_4$ cup diced avocado
		  $^1/_2$ cup mango salsa
		12 ounces grapefruit juice

2,800-CALORIES-PER-DAY MEAL PLAN OPTIONS
INTERVAL

ACTIVITY 3:00–5:00 p.m.	REBUILDING 5:00–8:00 p.m.	ANTI-STRESS 8:00–11:00 p.m.
100 51% 23% 26%	1080 25% 35% 40%	100 20% 80% 0%

1 stick light string cheese
3/4 cup cubed cantaloupe
	9 ounces top sirloin steak (lean), grilled
	  or broiled
	3/4 cup mashed potatoes*
	3/4 cup creamed spinach*
	1 ounce cheddar cheese
	1 ear corn on the cob
		4 ounces roasted
		  turkey breast

5 2-inch reduced-fat wheat crackers
1/2 ounce low-fat cheddar cheese
	Cheeseburger consisting of:
	  1 whole-wheat hamburger bun
	  8 ounces ground round beef
	  2 ounces mozzarella cheese
	  Pickles, onions, lettuce, tomato
	  1 cup steamed broccoli with 1 teaspoon
	  butter
	  16 ounces 1% milk
		3/4 cup fat-free
		  cottage cheese

1 1/2 ounces roasted chicken breast
3 ounces orange juice
	9 ounces braised pork rump roast
	1/2 cup cooked black beans, topped with
	  1 tablespoon sour cream
	1 cup steamed green beans
	1 slice cornbread (about 4- to 2-inch
	  square)
		2 scoops vanilla
		  whey protein
		  power
		  Water

	Spanish chicken consisting of:
	  9 ounces grilled chicken breast, seared
	  with 1 tablespoon olive oil
	  1 cup cooked black beans
	  2 ounces cheddar cheese
	  1/3 cup crushed tortilla strips	

	Sandwich consisting of:
	  2 slices whole-wheat bread
	  8 ounces turkey breast
	  4 slices Genoa salami
	  2 ounces cheddar cheese
	  1 tablespoon mayonnaise
	  1 1/4 cups fresh fruit cocktail	

* See page 177 for Mashed Potato and Creamed Spinach recipes

3,000-CALORIES-PER-DAY MEAL PLAN OPTIONS
INTERVAL

	RESTORATION 7:00–9:00 a.m.	ACTIVITY Noon–2:00 p.m.
Calories: **Carbohydrate:** **Protein:** **Fat:**	630 60% 20% 20%	1020 62% 7% 31%
Option 1	2 cups Cheerios or a comparable cereal 12 ounces 1% milk Fiber One bar $1/2$ cup strawberries $1 1/2$ sticks light string cheese	Large salad consisting of: 3 cups green leaf lettuce $1/2$ cup cooked black beans 1 cup corn $1/2$ cup diced onions 1 cup sliced bell pepper 1 cup halved cherry tomatoes $2 1/2$ tablespoons olive oil dressing with 1 tablespoon vinegar 2 slices whole-wheat bread 12 ounces grape juice
Option 2	1 cup cooked oatmeal Peanut butter toast consisting of: 2 slices whole-wheat toast 1 tablespoon peanut butter $1/2$ medium grapefruit Coffee with $1/2$ tablespoon fat-free French vanilla creamer $1/2$ cup low-fat cottage cheese 1 cup strawberries	$2/3$ cup hummus 1 whole-wheat pita pocket Small salad consisting of: 2 cups mixed salad greens $1/2$ cup diced avocado 1 tablespoon Italian dressing $1 1/4$ cups mixed, fresh berries 16 ounces pomegranate juice
Option 3	1 instant oatmeal packet with maple and brown sugar 2 slices whole-wheat toast 1 plum 1 whole large eggs with 1 large egg whites, scrambled 2 slices grilled Canadian bacon	Stuffed baked potato consisting of: 1 large baked potato 1 cup steamed broccoli 1 tablespoon butter 2 tablespoons sour cream 1 ounce honey-roasted cashews (about 18 nuts) 1 medium peach 16-ounce vegetable and fruit fusion drink
Option 4	2 eggs, cooked any style $1/2$ grapefruit $1/2$ cup low-fat granola $3/4$ cup fat-free, yogurt 8 ounces apple juice Breakfast taco consisting of: 2 corn tortillas	Eggplant pasta consisting of: $1 1/3$ cup cooked angel hair pasta 1 cup eggplant, sautéed with $1 1/4$ tablespoon olive oil, plus Italian herbs and garlic to taste $1 1/2$ cups blackberries 9 ounces pineapple juice 1 ounce honey-roasted cashews (about 18 nuts)
Option 5	1 large whole egg 1 ounce turkey sausage $1/2$ ounce cheddar cheese 12 ounces orange juice 1 large apple	Spaghetti consisting of: $1 1/3$ cup cooked spaghetti 1 cup spaghetti sauce 10 to 12 steamed asparagus spears with 1 tablespoon olive oil 8 ounces 1% milk 9 prunes

3,000-CALORIES-PER-DAY MEAL PLAN OPTIONS
INTERVAL

ACTIVITY 3:00–5:00 p.m.	REBUILDING 5:00–8:00 p.m.	ANTI-STRESS 8:00–11:00 p.m.
100 51% 23% 26%	1010 25% 35% 40%	100 20% 80% 0%
1 stick light string cheese $3/_4$ cup cubed cantaloupe	9 ounces top sirloin steak (lean), grilled or broiled $3/_4$ cup mashed potatoes* 1 ounce cheddar cheese $3/_4$ cup creamed spinach* $3/_4$ ear corn on the cob 4 ounces apple juice	4 ounces roasted turkey breast
5 2-inch reduced-fat wheat crackers $1/_2$ ounce low-fat cheddar cheese	Cheeseburger consisting of: 1 whole-wheat hamburger bun 7 ounces ground round beef 2 ounces mozzarella cheese Pickles, onions, lettuce, tomato $1/_2$ cup steamed broccoli with 1 teaspoon butter 16 ounces 1% milk	$3/_4$ cup fat-free cottage cheese
$1^1/_2$ ounces roasted chicken breast 3 ounces orange juice	8 ounces braised pork rump roast $1/_2$ cup cooked black beans 1 slice cornbread (about 4- to 2-inch square)	2 scoops vanilla whey protein power Water
	Spanish chicken consisting of: 8 ounces grilled chicken breast, seared with 1 tablespoon olive oil 1 cup cooked black beans 2 ounces cheddar cheese $1/_3$ cup crushed tortilla strips	
	Sandwich consisting of: 2 slices whole-wheat bread 7 ounces turkey breast 4 slices Genoa salami 2 ounces cheddar cheese 1 tablespoon mayonnaise $1^1/_4$ cups fresh fruit cocktail	

* See page 177 for Mashed Potato and Creamed Spinach recipes

5. SUPER-FUNCTIONAL FOODS

Following are five super-functional ingredients that should be part of your daily diet and the best food sources for them. These super-functional foods have a significant impact on helping you achieve your fitness goals, so whenever possible, include them in your daily diet. An important principle of the Hardwired Fitness Program is eating the right foods at the right time. Consuming foods that contain super-functional ingredients can deliver significant benefits in controlling appetite and increasing lean body mass. Table 11.6 also illustrates the best time to consume foods rich in specific super-functional ingredients.

Table 11.6. Super-Functional Ingredients

Super-functional Ingredients	Best Food Sources	Best Interval/Time to Consume Food
Branched-chain amino acids	Almonds, beef, chicken, chickpeas (garbanzo beans), eggs, lentils, milk, peanuts, salami/sausage, shrimp, soybeans, walnuts	Rebuilding: 5:00 P.M.–11:00 P.M.
Long-chain fatty acid	Almonds, avocados, cashews, grape seed oil, hazelnuts, macadamia nuts, olive oil, peanuts, pecans, pistachios, safflower oil, sesame oil, sunflower oil	Activity (later part): 3:00 P.M.–5:00 P.M.; Rebuilding: 5:00 P.M.–11:00 P.M.
B vitamin	Avocados, bananas, beef, cantaloupe, dairy products, eggs, fish, kiwifruits, nuts, oats, oranges, peaches, potatoes, poultry, tomatoes, watermelon, wheat bran, whole grains	Restoration: 7:00 A.M.–9:00 A.M.
Soluble fiber	Apples, apricots, bananas, blackberries, broccoli, brown rice, carrots, corn grits, grapefruits, green peas, lentils, oat bran, oranges, pears, pinto beans, plums, popcorn, potatoes, rolled oats, rye bread, squash (summer), strawberries, tangerines, zucchini	Restoration: 7:00 A.M.–9:00 A.M.; Activity (later part): 3:00 P.M.–5:00 P.M.; Rebuilding: 5:00 P.M.–11:00 P.M.

6. COMBINING LIFESTYLE ACTIVITY AND EXERCISE

One convenient way to increase energy expenditure and meet your threshold activity level is to add a little exercise while working at your desk. Exercising at your desk isn't as difficult as you might imagine. Actually, with a little imagination, you can find all kinds of ways to tone muscle and burn a few extra calories. Below are ten exercises that you can do while sitting at your desk. They will be a little difficult at first because you are probably not use to doing exercises in your chair. A little practice, however, and they will feel second nature. Completing this routine will increase your calorie expenditure by about 100 calories per day.

1. Toe raises—Sit up straight with your knees bent and your feet flat on the floor. Place your hands palms down on your knees. Raising both heels off the ground, shift the weight of your legs over your toes. Hold this position for 1 second, then lower your heels back to the ground. Repeat 20 times.

2. Hip flexions—Sit up straight with your knees bent and your feet flat on the floor. Lift one leg off the floor several inches, keeping both knees bent. Hold for 3 seconds, then lower your leg to the floor. Repeat 10 times and then switch legs.

3. Leg extensions—Sit up straight with your knees bent and your feet flat on the floor. Gradually extend one leg until it is parallel to the floor. Hold for 3 seconds, then lower the leg. Repeat 10 times and then switch legs.

4. Squats—Sit up straight with your knees bent and your feet flat on the floor. Holding your hands straight out in front with arms extended, come up off the chair without the use of your hands to about a half-standing position. Hold for 3 seconds, then lower yourself gently back down to a seated position. Repeat 10 times. Make sure the chair is secure and will not roll backward.

5. Dips—Sit up straight with your buttocks on the edge of the chair seat and your knees bent and your feet flat on the floor. Place your hands palms down on the chair seat beside your hips. Pressing your hands down, lift your buttocks off the seat. Now, lower your buttocks in front of and below the seat until your upper arms are just short of parallel to the floor. Repeat 10 times.

6. Bicep curls—Sit up straight with your knees bent and your feet flat on the floor. Place one hand palm down on your knee. Take a lightweight object such as a paperweight or a large bottle of water and hold it in your other hand with your arm down by your side. Now keeping the upper arm still, raise the weight upward by bending at the elbow. Raise the weight as high as possible without moving the upper arm and then lower the weight slowly and repeat 20 times. Repeat with the opposite arm.

7. Tricep curls—Sit up straight with your knees bent and your feet flat on the floor. Place one hand palm down on your knee. Holding a lightweight object in the other hand, raise it above your head with a straight arm. Now keeping the upper arm still, lower the weight backward by bending at the elbow. Once the weight has been lowered as far as possible, raise the weight back to a straight-arm position. Repeat 20 times then switch arms.

8. Arm presses—Sit up straight with your knees bent and your feet flat on the floor. Take a lightweight object in one hand and hold it beside your ear. Straightening your arm, raise the weight above your head and then lower your arm back into place. Repeat 15 times and then switch arms.

9. Crunches—Sit up straight with your knees bent and your feet flat on the floor. Clasp both hands together behind your head. Raise one knee to your chest while lowering your opposite elbow to the same knee and then lower knee and raise elbow. Alternate raising knees and lowering elbows and repeat and repeat 15 times with each knee.

10. Side pulls—Sit up straight with your knees bent and your feet flat on the floor. Turn your right shoulder 90 degrees toward your left side. Holding the chair arm or the side of the seat with your right hand, try to turn back to a normal sitting position using upper back muscles for 3 seconds. Repeat 8 times and then change sides.

It will take you about 15 minutes to do the full set of 10 exercises. However, you don't have to do all ten at once. You can do one or two at a time. Just be certain at the end of the day that you have completed all of them.

7. EXERCISE PROGRAMS

There is a wealth of information available on the web to help you select an exercise program that is right for you. Sites we highly recommend are listed in the Resources section of the tool kit on page 201. Here are examples of three excellent exercise programs.

Aerobic Exercise

Start your aerobic exercise by selecting an activity you enjoy doing and can do successfully for 30 minutes continuously at a moderate level of intensity. Walking, jogging, bicycling, swimming, exercising on fitness equipment, and cross-country skiing are a few of the many aerobic activities to pick from. Use your heart rate to determine your level of intensity. When starting out, your level of exercise intensity should be 60 percent of your heart rate reserve. Here is an easy way to determine your heart rate reserve:

1. Determine your maximum heart rate. Maximum heart rate can be estimated by subtracting your age from 220. So, if you are 42 years of age, your estimated maximum heart rate would be 178 beats per minute (220 − 42 = 178).

2. Next determine your resting heart rate. Sit quietly and place the tips of

your first two fingers of one hand on the bottom side of the opposite wrist just below the thumb. You should feel a strong pulse. Count the pulse beats for 15 seconds and multiply by 4. This will give your resting heart rate. As an example, let's assume it is 75 beats per minute.

3. Now use the following equation to calculate your heart rate reserve: (Maximum heart rate − resting heart rate) × .60 + resting heart rate = heart rate reserve. The heart rate reserve for our 42-year-old male would be: (178 − 75) × .60 + 75 = 137 beats per minute.

After six weeks of training, incorporate some interval training into your program. Interval training is exercising at different exercise intensities for short periods within your exercise session. For example, exercise for three minutes at an exercise intensity of 50 percent of your maximum heart rate and then one minute at 85 percent of maximum heart rate. This sequence would then be repeated eight times during a 32-minute workout session. Research has shown that interval workouts are the most effective means of bringing about a cardiovascular training response and it also appears to be a very efficient way to lose weight.

Put some variety into your exercise program. It is okay to jog on a treadmill one day, cycle the next and swim the third. A good game of racquetball, handball, or basketball thrown in would also be appropriate.

Resistance Exercise

Here are several things to keep in mind when beginning a resistance exercise program.

Start with light to moderate weights. This means weights that you can move easily through the full range of motion of the exercise; there should be no struggling with the movement. Resistance training exercises should be progressive in nature. This means that the exercise program should become more difficult as you become stronger. Your first workouts should not leave you with stiff, sore, achy muscles.

Design your program to work all the large muscles in the major areas of the body. These areas include the chest, back, shoulders, arms, legs, and abdominal region. Beginners should develop a program with 8 to 12 exercises with at least one exercise for each major body area.

Make sure you do the exercises you select correctly. Doing them incorrectly does not develop the muscles intended and may cause muscle pulls, strains, and possibly serious injury.

Make sure you complete a lift through its full range of motion.

Change up your exercise program every six to eight weeks. Gains in strength are very specific to how the muscle is being used, so it is good to train muscle groups with different exercises or movements.

Warm up before you start your resistance exercise workout. A good way to start is with about 5 to 10 minutes of cycling or walking on a treadmill, and then finish the warm-up with a few stretching exercises. This will help prevent any muscle pulls when you start your lifts.

Below are several exercises that can be performed at the gym for each of the six body regions that you will want to train. Select one or two exercises from each of the groups below. Do 10 to 12 repetitions per set, and plan to do your workout two to three days per week.

1. Chest—Dumbbell chest press, dumbbell chest fly, bench press

2. Shoulders—Lateral raise, front shoulder raise, upright row, shoulder press

3. Arms—Biceps curl, triceps kickback, triceps push-down using cable/ pulley system (on machine)

4. Back—Bent-over row, cable row, pull-down

5. Abdominal region—Abdominal crunch, side-knee crunches (pull knees up and to one side and crunch up)

6. Legs—Squats, leg extension (on machine), leg curl (on machine), and leg press (on machine)

Start out alternating upper body and lower body exercises. In the middle of your workout, do the abdominal exercises. Do exercises that use large muscles before exercises that use small muscles. For example, it would be better to do chest press exercises before doing tricep press-downs. With regard to time between exercises, one to two minutes is sufficient time if you are exercising to improve muscle tone and strength.

After two to three weeks of lifting, you should increase the number of sets per exercise to two, and allow about one to one and a half minutes of rest between sets. You may also want to increase the amount of weight you lift with each repetition.

Circuit Training Exercise

All you need to get started is a couple of light dumbbells (about 1 to 2 lbs each), a jump rope, and a watch with a second hand or stopwatch.

1. Warm up—Jog in place for 5 minutes.

2. Squat thrusts—Stand with your feet together. Squat down by shifting forward, and place your hands on the floor next to your feet. Now, jump your feet backward so you are in a push-up position, then jump your feet back between your hands and stand up. Do as many squat thrusts as you can in 10 seconds, rest for 5 seconds, and repeat four times.

3. Tricep kickbacks—Stand straight with your feet parallel and about hip-width apart. Bend at the waist until your back is straight and parallel to the floor. Holding a weight in each hand with your upper arms at your sides, bend your elbows, and bring the weights toward the rib cage, then straighten the elbows, squeezing the triceps (muscles in back of upper arm). Repeat for 1 minute.

4. Lunges with bicep curls—With the weights in your hands and standing with feet parallel and about hip-width apart, step forward with one foot bending at the knees so that the back knee almost touches the floor. At the same time, raise your hands to your chest by bending the arms at the elbows (bicep curls). Rise back up to standing position and lower your hands to your sides. Repeat for 1 minute, alternating legs.

5. Abdominal crunches—Lie on your back with your knees bent and your feet firmly on the floor. Fold your arms across your chest. Raise your head and shoulders off the floor about halfway to your knees. Hold for a count of 1. Lower your shoulders and head back toward the floor while maintaining tension in your abdominal muscles. Repeat for 1 minute.

6. Push-ups—Lie face down with your elbows bent and your hands on the floor at shoulder level. Legs should be straight back, feet together, with toes on the floor. Slowly push your body upward until your arms are straight. Then lower your body until your chest is just off the floor. Do not let your chest touch the floor. Your legs should remain straight and off the floor. However, if you find this too difficult, modify the push-up, by positioning yourself face down but on your hands and knees. Slowly straighten your elbows and push up off the floor until your arms are straight. Do as many push-ups as you can in 10 seconds, rest for 5 seconds, and repeat four times.

7. Back extensions—Lie face down with hands behind your head. Squeeze the lower back to lift your chest a few inches off the floor. Hold this position for a count of 2. Lower and repeat for 25 seconds. Rest for 10 seconds and repeat for 25 seconds.

8. Toe raises—Stand straight with your feet parallel and about hip-width apart. With arms by your sides and a weight in each hand, rise up on your toes. Hold this position for a count of 1 and then lower your heels to floor. Repeat for 1 minute.

9. Back raises with arm lifts—Stand straight with your feet parallel and about hip-width apart. With arms by your sides and a weight in each hand, bend slowly at the waist until your back is parallel with the floor while raising your hands with straight arms in front of your head. Hold for a count of 1. Lower your arms and repeat exercise for 1 minute.

10. Squats with shoulder press—Stand straight with your feet parallel and hip-width apart. Hold a weight in each hand at shoulder height with

your elbows pointed outward. Squat down by bending at your knees and keeping your back straight until your thighs are parallel with the floor. While squatting, raise (press) your hands up over your head and return to starting position. Repeat for 10 seconds and repeat the exercise for 25 seconds.

11. Lateral raises—Stand straight with your feet parallel and hip-width apart. Holding a weight in each hand down by your sides but with your elbows slightly bent, lift your arms out to your sides to shoulder level. Lower and repeat for 10 seconds. Rest for 5 seconds and repeat four times.

12. Jump rope—Jump rope continuously for 1 minute. Rest for 15 seconds. Repeat for 10 minutes.

13. Stretches—Cool down with 5 minutes of stretching.

When starting a circuit-training program, begin slowly, and rest when you need to. Gradually work to complete the exercise program as designed. Once you have mastered it, you can increase the intensity by increasing the time of each exercise and the weight that you are lifting.

8. HARDWIRED FITNESS SCORE WORKSHEET

You will be surprised at how rapidly you see changes in your fitness level. You will see changes in your weight and you will certainly notice changes in your body composition. However, the best way is to calculate your Hardwired Fitness Score (HFS) periodically. The first time it may seem a little tedious since you have to make a number of calculations; the next assessment will be much easier. By calculating your HFS, you will have a number with which to evaluate your progress. Directions for calculating each item are provided in Chapter 10.

HARDWIRED FITNESS SCORE WORKSHEET

NAME: _____ DATE: _____

WEEK 7: STARTING FITNESS LEVEL

1. BMI _____

2. % Body Fat _____

3. Net Activity Capacity (80 − Activity Capacity Value) _____

4. HFS (1 + 2 + 3) _____

WEEK 16: FITNESS LEVEL

1. BMI _____

2. % Body Fat _____

3. Net Activity Capacity (80 − Activity Capacity Value) _____

4. HFS (1 + 2 + 3) _____

WEEK 24: FITNESS LEVEL

1. BMI _____

2. % Body Fat _____

3. Net Activity Capacity (80 − Activity Capacity Value) _____

4. HFS (1 + 2 + 3) _____

HFS Score for Women

Age	Low Fit	Fit Range			High Fit
	Greater than	Moderately Low	Moderate	Moderately High	Less than
20–29	98	98–93	92–87	86–83	83
30–39	100	100–95	94–89	88–85	85
40–49	103	103–98	97–92	91–87	87
50–59	104	104–99	98–93	92–88	88
60+	107–102	101–96	95–91	91	91

HFS Score for Men

Age	Low Fit	Fit Range			High Fit
	Greater than	Moderately Low	Moderate	Moderately High	Less than
20–29	85	85–80	79–74	73–68	68
30–39	87	87–82	81–76	75–70	70
40–49	89	89–84	83–78	77–73	73
50–59	91	91–86	85–80	79–73	73
60+	94–89	88–84	83–76	76	76

9. RESOURCES

MEAL PLANNING

There are many excellent websites that can help you plan meals that are consistent with the core principles of Functional Eating. Many of these sites also have iPhone and BlackBerry applications available.

www.calorieking.com

www.diabetes.org/food-and-fitness

www.fitday.com

www.livestrong.com/thedailyplate

www.mypyramid.gov

www.nal.usda.gov/fnic/foodcomp/search

EXERCISE PROGRAMS

The following websites present an array of opportunities to get you moving. The offerings range from exercise routines and demos, DVDs and videos, finding a gym or trainer, and more.

www.active.com

www.crossfit.com

www.kettleball.com

www.fitnessmagazine.com

www.healthcentral.com/diet-exercise

www.livestrong.com

www.muscleandstrength.com/workouts

www.mypyramid.gov

www.shape.com

www.trainwithmeonline.com

Conclusion

The most important take-away message for anyone reading this book is how incredible the human body is. We have yet to create a machine that can function so efficiently over a wide range of environmental conditions, that can use multiple sources of fuel, that can repair itself and, if need be, even reprogram itself. In spite of this versatility and capacity, in a few short decades we have managed to impair the body's normal functioning. However, what this book hopefully has shown you is that it is not difficult to resynchronize your body. In doing so, you energize a powerful number of mechanisms to help you lose weight, increase lean body mass, and improve activity capacity. In writing this book, we were both amazed at finding research studies that not only confirmed the importance of the body's 24-hour functional rhythm, but that also showed once the body's biorhythms are resynchronized the force behind achieving a normal level of fitness is even stronger than we thought.

It is unfortunate that the contemporary mindset is to seek out magic bullets, whether they are nutritional programs or unusual exercise regimens. Each of them suggests that there is something wrong with your body that can only be corrected with the purchase of a book, device, food, or supplement. That is simply not the case. The evidence is overwhelming that within your DNA are powerful adaptive mechanisms that constantly push you to your normal state, which is one of fitness. All you have to do is respond naturally and let your body do its own thing.

References

Preface

Esmarck, B., Andersen, J.L., Olsen, S., et al. (2001) Timing of post-exercise protein intake is important for muscle hypertrophy with resistance training in elderly humans. *Journal of Physiology* 535: 301–311.

Ivy, J.L., Ding, Z., Hwang, H., et al. (2008) Post-exercise carbohydrate-protein supplementation: Phosphorylation of muscle proteins involved in glycogen synthesis and protein translation. *Amino Acids* 35: 89–97.

Volpi, E., Mittendorfer, B., Wolf, S.E. & Wolfe, R.R. (1999) Oral amino acids stimulate muscle protein anabolism in the elderly despite higher first-pass splanchnic extraction. *American Journal of Physiology—Endocrinology and Metabolism* 277: E513–E520.

Introduction

Associated Press. Dieting usually fails in the long run, study finds. April 2007.

Finkelstein, M.M. (Aug 2000) Body mass index and quality of life in a survey of primary care patients. *Journal of Family Practice* online. Retrieved from www.jfponline.com.

Mann, T., Tomiyama, A.J., Westling, E., et al. (2007) Medicare's search for effective obesity treatment. *American Psychologist* 62: 220–233.

Morbidity and Mortality Weekly Report (2007 Nov 23) Prevalence of regular physical activity among adults—United States, 2001 and 2005. *MMWR Publications* 56: 1209–1212. Retrieved from www.cdc.gov/mmwr.

Oz, M., and Roizen, M. If you're fit, does it matter if you're fat? *RealAge* online. Retrieved from www.realage.com.

Sheehan, T.J., DuBrava, S., DeChello, L.M., et al. (2003) Rates of weight change for black and white Americans over a twenty-year period. *International Journal of Obesity* 27: 498–504.

Chapter 1: Survival of the Fittest, Not the Thinnest

Blair, S.N., & Brodney, S. (1999) Effects of physical inactivity and obesity on morbidity and mortality: Current evidence and research issues. *Medicine and Science in Sports and Exercise* 31:, S646–S662.

Buchholz, A.C., & Schoeller, D.A. (2004) Is a calorie a calorie? *American Journal of Clinical Nutrition* 79: 899S–906S.

Centers for Disease Control. (1999 Nov17) Physical activity and health: A report of the surgeon general.

Centers for Disease Control. (2006) Prevalence of overweight and obesity among adults: United States, 2003–2004. www.cdc.gov/nchs/data/hestat/overweight/overweight_adult.htm.

Chong, D.L., Blair, S.N., & Jackson, A.S. (1999). Cardiorespiratory fitness, body composition, and all-cause and cardiovascular disease mortality in men. *American Journal of Clinical Nutrition* 69: 373–380.

Cutler, D.M., Glaeser, E.L., & Shapiro, J.M. (2003) Why have Americans become more obese? *Journal of Economic Perspectives* 17: 93–118.

Dimeo, F., Schwartz, S., Wesel, N., et al. (2008) Effects of an endurance and resistance exercise program on persistent cancer-related fatigue after treatment. *Annals of Oncology* 19: 1495–1499.

Feinman, R.D., & Fine, E.J. (2004) "A calorie is a calorie" violates the second law of thermodynamics. *Nutrition Journal* 3: 9.

Holloszy, J.O. (2005) Exercise-induced increase in muscle insulin sensitivity. *Journal of Applied Physiology*, 99: 338–343.

Ivy, J. & Portman, R. (2004) *Nutrient Timing* Basic Health Publications: North Bergen, NJ.

Kuczmarski, R.J., & Flegal, K.M. (2000) Criteria for definition of overweight in transition: Background and recommendations for the United States. *American Journal of Clinical Nutrition* 72: 1074–1081.

Manson, J.E., Hu, F.B., Rich-Edwards, J.W., et al. (1999) A prospective study of walking as compared with vigorous exercise in the prevention of coronary heart disease in women. *New England Journal of Medicine* 341: 650–658.

Myers, J., Prakash, M., Froelicher, V., et al. (2002) Exercise capacity and mortality among men referred for exercise testing. *New England Journal of Medicine* 346: 793–801.

Ogden, C.L., Fryar, C.D., Carroll, M.D., et al. (2004, Oct 27) Mean body weight, height, and body mass index, United States, 1960–2002. CDC Advance Data from Vital and Health Statistics, Number 347.

Peschke, E., & Peschke, D. (1998) Evidence for a circadian rhythm of insulin release from perifused rat pancreatic islets. *Diabetologia* 41: 1085–1092.

Speakman, J.R. (2007 Jul) A nonadaptive scenario explaining the genetic predisposition to obesity: The "predation release" hypothesis. *Cell Metabolism* 6: 5–12.

Stubbs, R.J., Hughes, D.A., Johnstone, A.M., et al. (2004) A decrease in physical activity affects appetite, energy, and nutrient balance in lean men feeding ad libitum. *American Journal of Clinical Nutrition* 79: 62–69.

Sui X., LaMonte M.J., Laditka, J.N., et al. (2007 Dec 5) Cardiorespiratory fitness and adiposity as mortality predictors in older adults. *Journal of the American Medical Association* 298: 2507–2516.

Szabo, A. (2003) Acute psychological benefits of exercise performed at self-selected workload: Implications for theory and practice. *Journal of Sports Science and Medicine* 2: 77–87.

Warburton, D.E.R., Nicol, C.W., & Bredin, S.S.D. (2006) Health benefits of physical activity: the evidence. *Canadian Medical Association Journal*, 174: 801–809.

Wei, M., Kampert, J.B., Barlow, C.E., et al. (1999) Relationship between low cardiorespiratory fitness and mortality in normal-weight, overweight and obese men. *Journal of the American Medical Association* 282: 1547–53.

Williamson, D.F., Kahn, H., Remington, P.L., et al. (1990) The 10-year incidence of overweight and major weight gain in US adults. *Archives of Internal Medicine* 150: 665–672.

Chapter 2: Circuits and Rhythms

American Physiological Society. (2008 Dec 12) Aerobic exercise stimulates release of appetite suppressing hormone. Online article in *Exercise, Weight and Obesity*. Retrieved from www.worldhealth.net/news/aerobic_exercise_stimulates_release_of_a.

Bjorntorp P. (2001) Do stress reactions cause abdominal obesity and comorbidities? *Obesity Reviews* 2: 73–86.

Blair, S.N., & Brodney, S. (1999) Effect of physical inactivity and obesity on morbidity and mortality: Current evidence and research issues. *Medicine and Science in Sports and Exercise* 31: S646–S662.

Carling, D. (2005) Amp-activated protein kinase: balancing the scales. *Biodhimie*, 87: 87_91.

Cheng, M.H., Bushnell, D., Cannon, D.T., et al. (2009) Appetite regulation via exercise prior or subsequence to high-fat meal consumption. *Appetite* 52: 193–198.

Cota, D., Proulx, K., Blake Smith, K.A., et al. (2006) Hypothalamic mTor signaling regulates food intake. *Science* 312: 927–930.

Cotton, J.R., Burley, V.J., Weststrate, J.A., et al. (1994) Dietary fat and appetite: similarities and differences in the satiating effects of meals supplemented with either fat or carbohydrate. *Journal of Human Nutrition and Dietetics* 7: 11–24.

Dansinger, M.L., Gleason, J.A., Griffith, J.L., et al. (2005) Comparison of the Atkins, Ornish, Weight Watchers and Zone Diets for weight loss and heart disease risk reduction: A randomized trial. *Journal of the American Medicine Association* 293: 43–53.

Lee, C.D., Blair, S.N., & Jackson, A.S. (1999) Cardiorespiratory fitness, body composition, and all-cause and cardiovascular disease mortality in men. *American Journal of Clinical Nutrition* 69: 373–380.

Maglione-Garves, C., Kravitz, L., & Schneider, S. (2005) Cortisol connection: Tips on managing stress and weight. American College of Sports Medicine's *Health & Fitness Journal* 9(5): 20–23.

Martins, C., Morgan, L.M., & Truby, H. (2008) A review of the effects of appetite regulation: an obesity perspective. *International Journal of Obesity*, 32: 1337–1347.

Matsakas, A. & Patel, K. (2009) Intercellular signalling pathways regulating the adaptation of skeletal muscle to exercise and nutritional changes. *Histology and Histopathology*, 24: 209–222.

Medical News Today Online (2007 Dec 5) Fit over 60s live longer regardless of body fat. Retrieved from www.medicalnewstoday.com/articles/90705.php.

Merchant, A.T., Vatanparast, H., Barlas, S., et al. (2009) Carbohydrate intake and overweight and obesity among healthy adults. *Journal of the American Dietetic Association* 109: 1165–1172.

Minokoshi, Y., Shiuchi, T., Lee, S., et al. (2008) Role of hypothalamic AMP-kinase in food intake regulation. *Nutrition*, 24: 786–790.

Myers, J., Kaykha, A., George, S., et al. (2004) Fitness versus physical activity patterns in predicting mortality in men. *American Journal of Medicine* 117: 912–918.

Ohkawara, K., Tanaka, S., Ishikawa-Takata, K., et al. (2008) Twenty-four-hour analysis of elevated energy expenditure after physical activity in a metabolic chamber: Models of daily total energy expenditure. *American Journal of Clinical Nutrition* 87: 1268–1276.

Piomelli, D., et al. (2008) The lipid messenger OEA links dietary fat intake to satiety. *Cell Metabolism* 8: 281–288.

Sagara, T., Hitomi, Y., Kambayashi, Y., et al. (2009) Common risk factors for changes in body weight and psychological well-being in Japanese male middle-aged workers. *Environmental Health and Preventive Medicine*, 14: 319–327.

Wei, M., Kampert, J.B., Barlow, C.E., et al. (1999) Relationship between low cardiorespiratory fitness and mortality in normal-weight, overweight and obese men. *Journal of the American Medical Association* 27: 1547–1553.

Woo, R., Garrow, J.S., Pi-Sunyer, F.X. (1982) Effect of exercise on spontaneous calorie intake in obesity. *American Journal of Clinical Nutrition* 36: 470–447.

Woods, S.C., Seeley, R.J., Porte, D., et al. (1998) Signals that regulate food intake and energy homeostasis. *Science* 280: 1378–1383.

Chapter 3: High-Speed Communication Network

Blundell, J.E., Stubbs, R.J., Hughes, D.A., et al. (2003) Cross talk between physical activity and appetite control: does physical activity stimulate appetite? *Procedings of the Nutrition Society*, 62: 651–661.

Broom, D.R., Batterham, R.L., King, J.A., et al. (2009) Influence of resistance and aerobic exercise on hunger, circulating levels of acylated ghrelin, and peptide YY in healthy males. *American Journal of Physiology-Regulatory Integrative and Comparative Physiology*, 296: R29–R35.

Carling, D. (2005) Amp-activated protein kinase: balancing the scales. *Biohimie*, 87: 87–91.

Coccurello, R., d'Amato, F.R., & Moles, A. (2009) Chronic social stress, hedonism and vulnerability to obesity: Lessons learned from rodents. *Neuroscience and Biobehavioral Reviews*, 33: 537–550.

Cota, D., Proulx, K., Smith, K.A.B., et al. (2006) Hypothalamic mTOR signaling regulates food intake. *Science*, 312, 927–930.

Froy, O. (2007) The relationship between nutrition and circadian rhythms in mammals. *Frontiers in Neuroendocrinology*, 28: 61–71.

Ivy, J.L., Ding, Z., Hwang, H., et al. (2008) Post exercise carbohydrate-protein supplementation: phosphorylation of muscle protein involved in glycogen synthesis and protein translation. *Amino Acids*, 32: 381–386

Inoki, K., Ouyang, H., Li, Y., et al. (2005) Signaling by target of rapamycin proteins in cell growth control. *Microbiology and Molecular Biology Reviews*, 69: 79–100.

Norton, L.E. & Layman, D.K. (2006) Leucine regulates translation of protein synthesis in skeletal muscle after exercise. *Journal of Nutrition*, 136: S533–S537.

Martins, C., Morgan, L.M., Bloom, S.R., et al. (2007) Effects of exercise on gut peptides, energy intake and appetite. *Journal of Endocrinology*, 193: 251–258.

Martins, C., Morgan, L.R. & H. Truby. (2008) A review of the effects of appetite regulation: an obesity perspective. *International Journal of Obesity*, 32: 1337–1347.

Matsakas, A. & Patel, K. (2009) Intercellular signaling pathways regulating the adaptation of skeletal muscle to exercise and nutritional changes. *Histology and Histopathology*, 24: 209–222.

Minokoshi, Y., Shiuchi, T., Lee, S., et al. (2008) Role of hypothalamic AMP-kinase in food intake regulation. *Nutrition*, 24: 786–790.

Morrison, P.J., Hara, D., Ding, Z., & Ivy, J.L. (2008) Providing nutrients after endurance exercise stimulates mRNA translation signaling pathways in rats. *Journal of Applied Physiology*, 104: 1029–1036.

Nieuwenhuizen, A.G. & Rutters, F. (2008) The hypothalamic-pituitary-adrenal-axis in the regulation of energy balance. *Physiology and Behavior*, 94: 169–177.

Proud, C.G. (2004) mTOR-mediated regulation of translation factors by amino acids. *Biochemical and Biophysical Research Communications*, 313: 429–436.

Obici, S. & Rossetti, L. (2003) Minireview: Nutrient sensing and the regulation of insulin action and energy balance. *Endocrinology*, 144: 5172–5178

Ramsey, K.M., Marcheva, B., Kohsaka, A., et al. (2007) The clockwork of metabolism. *Annual Review of Nutrition*, 27: 219–240.

Sagara, T., Hitomi, Y., Kambayashi, Y., et al. (2009) Common risk factors for changes in body weight and psychological well-being in Japanese male middle-aged workers. *Environmental Health and Preventive Medicine*, 14: 319–327.

Sakamoto, K., Aschenbach, W.G., Hirshman, M.F., et al. (2003) Akt signaling in skeletal muscle: regulation by exercise and passive stretch. *American Journal of Physiology-Endocrinology and Metabolism*, 285: E1081–E1081.

Sriwijitkamol, A., Ivy, J.L., Christ-Roberts, C., et al. (2006) LKB1-AMPK signaling in muscle from obese insulin resistant Zucker rats and effects of training. *American Journal of Physiology-Endocrinology and Metabolism*, 290: E925–E932.

Chapter 4: Disconnected and Overloaded Circuits

Apfelbaum, M., Bostsarron, J., & Lacatis, D. (1971) Effect of caloric restriction and excessive caloric intake on energy expenditure. *American Journal of Clinical Nutrition* 24: 1405–1409.

Associated Press. Sleep deprivation raises obesity risk, study finds. *St. Petersburg Times Online*, Nov17, 2004. Retrieved from www.sptimes.com/2004/11/17/Worldandnation/Sleep_deprivation_rai.shtml.

Ball, M.F., Kyle, L.H., & Canary, J.J. (1967) Comparative effects of caloric restriction and metabolic acceleration on body composition in obesity. *Journal of Clinical Endocrinology & Metabolism*, 27: 273–278.

Ballor, D.L., Katch, V.L., Becque, M.D., et al. (1988) Resistance weight training during caloric restriction enhances lean body weight maintenance. *American Journal of Clinical Nutrition* 47: 19–25.

Blundell, J.E., Stubbs, R.J., Hughes, D.A., et al. (2003) Cross talk between physical activity and appetite control: does physical activity stimulate appetite? *Proceedings of the Nutrition Society* 62: 651–661.

Brownell, K.D., Greenwood, M.R.C., Stellar, E., et al. (1986) The effects of repeated cycles of weight loss and regain in rats. *Physiology & Behavior* 38: 459–464.

Das, S.K., Saltzman, E., Gilhooly, C.H., et al. (2009 Apr 23) Low or moderate dietary energy restriction for long-term weight loss: What works best? *Obesity* online. Retrieved from www.nature.com/oby/journal/vaop/ncurrent/abs/oby2009120a.html.

Durrant, M.L., Garrow, J.S., Royston, P., et al. (1980) Factors influencing the composition of the weight lost by obese patients on a reducing diet. *British Journal of Nutrition* 44(3): 275–285.

Farshchi, H.R., Taylor, M.A., & and Macdonald, I.A. (2004) Regular meal frequency creates more appropriate insulin sensitivity and lipid profiles compared with irregular meal frequency in healthy lean women. *European Journal of Clinical Nutrition* 58: 1071–1077.

Gardner, D.S., & Rhodes, P. (2009) Developmental origins of obesity: Programming of food intake or physical activity? *Advances in Experimental Medicine and Biology* 646: 83–93.

Hill, A.J. (2004) Does dieting make you fat? *British Journal of Nutrition* 92: S15–S18.

Hill, J.O., Wyatt, H.R., Reed, G.W., et al. (2003) Obesity and the environment: Where do we go from here? *Science* 299: 853–855.

Leibel, R.L., Rosenbaum, M., & Hirsch, J. (1995) Changes in energy expenditure resulting from altered body weight. *New England Journal of Medicine* 332: 621–628.

Lenard, N.R., & Berthoud, H.R. (2008) Central and peripheral regulation of food intake and physical activity: Pathways and genes. *Obesity* 16: S11–S22.

Leproult, R., Copinschi, G., Buxton, O., et al. (1997) Sleep loss results in an elevation of cortisol levels the next evening. *Journal of Sleep Research and Sleep Medicine* 20(10): 865–870.

Lim, K., Murakami, E., Lee, S., et al. (1996 Oct) Effects of intermittent food restriction and refeeding on energy efficiency and body fat deposition in sedentary and exercised rats. *Journal of Nutritional Science and Vitaminology* 42(5): 449–468.

Manore, M.M., Berry, T.E., Skinner, J.S., et al. (1991) Energy expenditure at rest and during exercise in nonobese female cyclical dieters and in nondieting control subject. *American Journal of Clinical Nutrition* 54: 41–46.

Mayer, J., Roy, P., & Mitra, K.P. (1956) Relationship between caloric intake, body weight, and physical work: Studies in industrial male population in West Bengal. *American Journal of Clinical Nutrition* 4: 169.

Montani, J.P., Viecelli, A.K., Prevot, A., et al. (2006) Weight cycling during growth and beyond as a risk factor for later cardiovascular diseases: The "repeated overshoot" theory. *International Journal of Obesity*, 30: S58–S66.

Ravussin, E., Burnand, B., Schutz, Y., et al. (1985) Energy expenditure before and during energy restriction in obese patients. *American Journal of Clinical Nutrition* 41: 753–759.

Reuters. Sleep deprivation tied to weight gain. June 10, 2009.

Spiegel, K., Knutson, K., Leproult, R., et al. (2005) Sleep loss: A novel risk factor insulin resistance in type 2 diabetes. *Journal of Applied Physiology* 99: 2008–2019.

Stote, K.S., Baer, D.J., Spears, K., et al. (2007) A controlled trial of reduced meal fre-quency without caloric restriction in healthy, normal-weight, middle-aged adults. *American Journal of Clinical Nutrition* 85: 981–988.

Taheri, S., Lin, L., Austin, D., et al. (2004) Short sleep duration is associated with reduced leptin, elevated ghrelin, and increased body mass index. *PLos Med* 1(3): e62.

Van Cauter, E., Knutson, K., Leproult, R., et al. The impact of sleep deprivation on hormones and metabolism. *Medscape Neurology & Neurosurgery.* April 28, 2005. Retrieved from http://cme.medscape.com/viewarticle/502825?rss.

Warren, T.Y., Vaughn, B., Hooker, S.P., et al. (2010) Sedentary Behaviors Increase Risk of Cardiovascular Disease Mortality in Men. *Medicine & Science in Sports & Exer-cise* 42(5): 879–885.

Yanovski, J.A., Yanovski, S.Z., Sovik, K.N., et al. (2000) A prospective study of holiday weight gain. *New England Journal of Medicine* 342: 861–867.

Chapter 5: Resynchronizing and Resetting the Circuits

Blundell, J.E., & King, N.A. (1999) Physical activity and regulation of food intake: Current evidence. *Medicine and Science in Sport and Exercise* 31: S573–S583.

Hamilton, M.T., Hamilton, D.G., & Zderic, T.W. (2007) Role of low energy expendi-ture and sitting in obesity, metabolic syndrome, type 2 diabetes, and cardiovascular dis-ease. *Diabetes* 56: 2655–2667.

Katzmarzyk, P.T., Church, T.S., Craig, C.L., et al. (2009) Sitting time and mortality from all causes, cardiovascular disease, and cancer. *Medicine and Science in Sports and Exercise* 41(5): 998–1005.

Levine, J.A., Schleusner, S.J., & Jensen, M.D. (2000) Energy expenditure of nonexer-cise activity. *American Journal of Clinical Nutrition* 72: 1451–1454.

Levine, J.A., Vander Weg, M.W., Hill, J.O., et al. (2006) Non-exercise activity thermo-genesis: The crouching tiger hidden dragon of societal weight gain. *Arteriosclerosis, Thrombosis and Vascular Biology* 26: 729–736.

Stubbs, R.J., Hughes, D.A., Johnston, A.M., et al. (2004) A decrease in physical activi-ty affects appetite, energy, and nutritional balance in lean men feeding ad libitum. *American Journal of Nutrition* 79: 62–69.

Chapter 6: The Functional Day

ABC News Poll. (2005 May 17) What Americans eat for breakfast. Retrieved from http://abcnews.go.com/gma/pollvault/story?id=762685.

Bellisle, F., McDevitt, R., & Prentice A. (1997) Meal frequency and energy balance. *British Journal of Nutrition* 77: S57–S70.

Bennard, P., & Doucet, E. (2006) Acute effects of exercise timing and breakfast meal glycemic index on exercise-induced fat oxidation. *Applied Physiology, Nutrition, and Metabolism* 31: 501–511.

Berg, C., Lappas, G., & Wolk, A. (2009) Eating patterns and portion size associated with obesity in a Swedish population. *Appetite* 52(1): 21–26.

Bertéus Forslund, H., Lindroos, A.K., Sjostrom, L., et al. (2002) Meal patterns and obesity in Swedish women: A simple instrument describing usual meal types, frequency and temporal distribution. *European Journal of Clinical Nutrition* 56: 740–747.

Blom, W.A., Lluch, A., Stafleu, A., et al. (2006) Effect of a high-protein breakfast on the postpradial ghrelin response. *American Journal of Clinical Nutrition* 84: 664–665.

Blundell, J.E., Stubbs, R.J., Hughes, D.A., et al. (2003) Cross talk between physical activity and appetite control: Does physical activity stimulate appetite? *Proceedings of the Nutrition Society* 62: 651–661.

Camire, M.E., & Blackmore, M. (2007) Breakfast foods and satiety. *Food Technology* 61(2): 24–30.

Castiglione, K.E., Read, N.W., & French, S.J. (2002) Adaptation to high-fat diet accelerated emptying of fat but not carbohydrate test meals in humans. *American Journal of Physiology-Regulatory, Integrative and Comparative Physiology* 282: R366–R371.

Chapelot, D., Marmonier, C., Aubert, R.P., et al. (2006) Consequence of omitting or adding a meal in man on body composition, food intake and metabolism. *Obesity* 14: 215–227.

De Castro, J.M. (1987) Circadian rhythms of the spontaneous meal pattern, macronutrient intake, and the mood of humans. *Physiology and Behavior* 40: 427–446.

De Castro, J.M. (2004 Jan) The time of day of food intake influences overall intake in humans. *Journal of Clinical Nutrition* 134: 104–111.

De Castro, J.M. (2007) The time of day and the proportions of macronutrients eaten are related to total daily intake. *British Journal of Nutrition* 98: 1077–1083.

Drummond, S.E., Cromble, N.E., Cursiter, M.C., et al. (1998) Evidence that eating frequency is inversely related to body weight status in male, but not female, non-obese adults reporting valid dietary intake. *Journal of the International Association for the Study of Obesity* 22: 105–112.

Eng, S., Wagstaff, D.A., & Kranz, S. (2009) Eating late in the evening is associated with childhood obesity in some age groups but not in all children: The relationship between time of consumption and body weight status in U.S. children. *International Journal of Behavioral Nutrition and Physical Activity* 6: 27.

Forslund, A.H., El-Khoury, A. E., Olsson, R. M., et al. (1999) Effect of protein intake and physical activity on 24-h pattern and rate of macronutrient utilization. *Journal of the American Physiological Society:* E964–E976.

Fox News. (2008 June 18) Big, carb-heavy breakfast key to weight loss. *Sky News.* Retrieved from http://www.foxnews.com/story/0,2933,368462,00.html.

Gardner, D.S., & Rhodes, P. (2009) Developmental origins of obesity: Programming of food intake or physical activity. *Advances in Experimental Medicine and Biology* 646: 83–93.

Gluck, M.E., Venti, C.A., Salbe, A.D., et al. (2008) Nighttime eating: Commonly observed and related to weight gain in an inpatient food intake study. *American Journal of Clinical Nutrition* 88: 900–905.

Hamilton, M.T., Hamilton, D.G., & Zderic, T.W. (2007) Role of low energy expenditure and sitting in obesity metabolic syndrome, type 2 diabetes, and cardiovascular disease. *Diabetes* 56: 2655–2667.

Haus, E. (2007) Chronobiology in the endocrine system. *Advanced Drug Delivery Reviews* 59: 985–1014.

Ishida, N., Miyazaki, K., & Sakai, T. (2001) Circadian rhythm biochemistry: From protein degradation to sleep and mating. *Biochemical and Biophysical Research Communications* 286: 1–5.

Jakubowicz, D. (2008 Jun 17) Study supports wisdom of big breakfast. Presented at the Endocrine Society 90th annual meeting in San Francisco.

Jones, P.J., Namchuk, G.L., & Pederson, R.A. (1995) Meal frequency influences circulating hormone levels but not lipogenesis rates in humans. *Metabolism* 44: 218–223.

Levine, A.S., Tallman, J.R., Grace, M.K., et al. (1989) Effect of breakfast cereals on short-term food intake. *American Journal of Clinical Nutrition* 50: 1303–1307.

Ma, Y., Bertone, E.R., Stanek, E.J., et al. (2003) Association between eating patterns and obesity in a free-living U.S. adult population. *American Journal of Epidemiology* 158: 85–92.

Mathews, C.E., Freedson, P.S., Herbert, J.R., et al. (2001) Seasonal variation in household, occupational, and leisure time physical activity: Longitudinal analyses from the seasonal variation of blood cholesterol study. *Journal of Epidemiology* 153: 172–183.

Matney, K. (2005 Spring) Circadian rhythms in shift workers and diabetes. Retrieved from http://serendip.brynmawr.edu/bb/neuro/neuro05/web3/kmatney.html.

Metzner, H.L., Lamphier, D.E., Wheeler, N.C., et al. (1977) The relationship between frequency of eating and adiposity in adult men and women in the Tecumseh Community Health Study. *American Journal of Clinical Nutrition* 30: 712–715.

Pasman, W.J., Blokdijk, V.M., Bertina, F.M., et al. (2003) Effect of two breakfasts, different in carbohydrate composition, on hunger and satiety and mood in healthy men. *International Journal of Obesity* 27: 663–668.

Salbe, A.D., Tschop, M.H., DelParigi, A., et al. (2004) Negative relationship between fasting plasma ghrelin concentration and *ad libitum* food intake. *Journal of Clinical Endocrinology & Metabolism* 89(6): 2951–2956.

Schlundt, D.G., Hill, J.O., Sbrocco, T., et al. (1992) The role of breakfast in the treatment of obesity: A randomized clinical trial. *American Journal of Clinical Nutrition* 55: 645–651.

Simon, C., Weibel, L., & Brandenberger, G. (2000) Twenty-four-hour rhythms of plasma glucose and insulin secretion rate in regular night workers. *American Journal of Physiology—Endocrinology and Metabolism* 278: E413–E420.

Smeets, A.J., Westerterp-Plantegna, M.S. (2008) Acute effect on metabolism and appetite profile of one meal difference in the lower range of meal frequency. *British Journal of Nutrition* 99: 1316–1321.

Solomon, T.P.J., Chambers, E.S., Jeukendrup, A.E., et al. (2008) The effect of feeding frequency on insulin and ghrelin responses in human subjects. *British Journal of Nutrition* 100: 810–819.

Van Der Heijden, A., Hu, F.B. Rimm, R.B., et al. (2007) A prospective study of breakfast consumption and weight gain among U.S. men. *Obesity* 15: 2463–2466.

Veldhorst, M.A., Nieuwenhuizen, A.G., Hochstenbach-Waelen, A., et al. (2008) Comparison of the effects of a high- and normal-casein breakfast on satiety, "satiety" hormone, plasma amino acids and subsequent energy intake. *British Journal of Nutrition* 18: 1–9.

Völkl, A. (1983) Circadian rhythm of protein synthesis activity in the exocrine pancreas of fed and starved rats. *Journal of Cell Science* 61: 467–473.

Westerterp-Plantenga, M.S., Kovacs, E.M.R., & Melanson, K.J. (2002) Habitual meal frequency and energy intake regulation in partially temporally isolated men. *International Journal of Obesity* 26: 102–110.

Winget, C.M., DeRoshia, C.W., & Holley, D.C. (1985) Circadian rhythms and athletic performance. *Medicine and Science in Sports and Exercise* 17: 498–515.

Young, V.R., & El-Khoury, A.E. (1996, Sept) Recent 24-hour tracer studies of amino acid requirements. In Human amino acid requirements: A re-evaluation. *Food and Nutrition Bulletin* 17: 3. Retrieved from www.unu.edu/unupress/food/8F173e/8F173E00.htm

Yunsheng, M., Bertone, E.R., Stanek, E.J., et al. (2003) Association between eating patterns and obesity in a free-living US adult population. *American Journal of Epidemiology* 158: 85–92.

Chapter 9: Switch Your Body into Fitness Mode

Aahahl, M., Kjaer, M., & Jørgensen, T. (2007) Perceived exertion of physical activity:

Negative association with self-related fitness. *Scandinavian Journal of Public Health* 35: 403–409.

Angevaren, M., Aufdemkampe, G., Verhaar, H.J., et al. (2008) Physical activity and enhanced fitness to improve cognitive function in older people without known cognitive impairment. Cochran Database Systems Review. CD005381.

Biener, L., & Heaton, A. (1995) Women dieters of normal weight: Their motives, goals and risks. *American Journal of Public Health* 85: 714–717.

Bishop, N.C. & Gleeson, M. (2009) Acute and chronic effects of exercise on markers of mucosal immunity. *Frontiers in Bioscience*, 14: 4444–4456.

Blair, S.N. & Connelly, J.C. (1996) How much physical activity should we do? The case for moderate amounts and intensities of physical activity. *Research Quarterly for Exercise and Sport*, 67: 193–205.

Blair, S.N., Kohl, H.W., Paffenbarger, R.S., et al. (1989) Physical fitness and all-cause mortality: A prospective study of healthy men and women. *Journal of the American Medical Association*, 262: 2395–2401.

Blair, S.N., LaMonte, M.J., & Nichaman, M.Z. (2004) The evolution of physical activity recommendations: How much is enough? *American Journal of Clinical Nutrition*, 79: 913S–920S.

Cloud, J. (2009 Aug 9) Why exercise won't make you thin. *Time* magazine.

Cooper, C.J. (1973) Anatomical and physiological mechanisms of arousal, with special reference to the effects of exercise. *Ergonomics*, 16: 601–609.

Holloszy, J.O. (2005) Exercise-induced increase in muscle insulin sensitivity. *Journal of Applied Physiology*, 99: 338–343.

Holmes, M.D., Chen, W.Y., Feskanich, D., et al. (2004) Physical activity in cancer survivors: Implications for recurrence and mortality. *Cancer Therapy*, 2: 1–12.

Honokola, A., Forsen, T. & Eriksson, J. (1997) Resistance training improves the metabolic profile in individuals with type 2 diabetes. *Acta Diabetologica*, 34: 245–248.

Ivy, J. & Portman, R. *Nutrient Timing*. Basic Health Publications, Inc. North Bergen, NJ. 2004.

Ivy, J., Zderic, T.W., & and Fogt, D.L. (1999) Prevention and treatment of NIDDM with exercise training. In: Exercise and Sports Science Reviews. Vol. 27, (Ed.) J.O. Holloszy, Williams & Wilkins, Baltimore, MD: 1–35.

Jackson, D. (2004 May) The effects of stress on exercise. *Personal Fitness Professional*. Retrieved from www.south-florida-personal-trainer.com/stress.html.

Koji, K., Maruyama, T., Murota, M., et al. (2009) Positive effects of acute and moderate physical exercise on cognitive function. *Journal of Physiological Anthropology*, 28: 155–164.

Kramer, A.F., Erickson, K.I. & Colcombe, S.J. (2006) Exercise, cognition, and the aging brain. *Journal of Applied Physiology* 101: 1237–1242.

Lakka, T.A. & Laaksonen, D.E. (2007) Physical activity in prevention and treatment of the metabolic syndrome. *Applied Physiology, Nutrition and Metabolism*, 32: 76–88.

Levenhagen, D.K., Carr, C., Carlson, M.G., et al. (2001) Postexercise protein intake enhances whole-body and leg protein accretion in humans. *Medicine and Science in Sports and Exercise* 34: 828–837.

Manson, J.E., Hu, F.B., Rich-Edwards, J.W., et al. (1999) A prospective study of walking as compared with vigorous exercise in the prevention of coronary heart disease in women. *New England Journal of Medicine*, 341: 650–658.

Mardian, J. (2009 Aug 3) The psychological benefits of exercise: Is it all in the head? *Health in Motion.* Retrieved from http://healthinmotion.wordpress.com/2009/08/03/the-psychological-benefits-of-exercise-is-it-all-in-the-head/.

Miller S.L., Tipton, K.D., Wolf, S.E., et al. (2003) Independent and combined effects of amino acids and glucose after resistance exercise. *Medicine and Science in Sports and Exercise* 35(3): 449–455.

Nakamura, Y., Nishimoto, K., Akamatu, M., et al. (1999) The effect of jogging on P300 event related potentials. *Electromyography and Clinical Neurophysiology*, 39: 71–74.

Northoff, H. Exercise immunology review. (2009) *Exercise Immunology Review*, 15: 5.

Norton, L., & Layman, D.K. (2006) Leucine regulates translation initiation of protein synthesis in skeletal muscle after exercise. *American Journal of Nutrition*, 136: 533S–537S.

Paez, C.J., & Kravitz, L. (2000) Exercise vs. diet in weight loss. *Exercise and Sport Science Reviews* 28: 165–170.

Paffenbarger, R.S., Jr., Hyde, R.T., Wing, A.L., et al. (1986) Physical activity, all-cause mortality, and longevity of college alumni. *New England Journal of Medicine*, 314: 605–613.

Paffenbarger, R.S., Jr., Lee, I.M., & Wing, A.L. (1992) The influence of physical activity on the incidence of site-specific cancers in college alumni. *Advances in Experimental Medicine and Biology*, 322: 7–15.

Quinn, E. (2007 Oct 29) Exercise and immunity: How moderate exercise boosts the immune system. *About.com.* Retrieved from http://sportsmedicine.about.com/cs/injuryprevention/a/aa011502a.htm.

Rhodes, R.E. & Fiala, B. (2009) Building motivation and sustainability into the prescription and recommendations for physical activity and exercise therapy: the evidence. *Physiotherapy Theory and Practice*, 25: 424–441.

Rippe, J. M. & Hess, S. (1998) The role of physical activity in the prevention and management of obesity. *Journal of American Dietetic Association*, 98: S31–S38.

Salmon, J., Booth, M.L., Phongsavan, P., et al. (2007) Promoting physical activity participation among children and adolescents. *Epidemiological Review*, 29: 144–159, 2007.

Stiegler, P. & Cunliffe, A. (2006) The role of diet and exercise for the maintenance of fat-free mass and resting metabolic rate during weight loss. *Sports Medicine*, 36: 239–262.

Stofan, J.R., DiPietro, L., Davis, D., et al. (1998) Physical activity patterns associated with cardiorespiratory fitness and reduced mortality: The aerobics center longitudinal study. *American Journal of Public Health*, 88: 1807–1813.

Thune, I., & Furberg, A.S. (2001) Physical activity and cancer risk: dose-response and cancer, all sites and site-specific. *Medicine and Science in Sport and Exercise*, 33: S530–S550.

Tuomilehto, J., Lindstrom, J., Eriksson, J.G., et al. (2001) Prevention of type 2 diabetes mellitus by changes in lifestyle among subjects with impaired glucose tolerance. *New England Journal of Medicine*, 344: 1343–1350.

Wang, X., Lyles, M.F., You T., et al. (2008) Weight regain is related to decreases in physical activity during weight loss. *Medicine and Science in Sports and Exercise* 40: 1781–1788.

Warburton, D.E., Gledhill, N., & Quinney, A. (2001) Musculoskeletal fitness and health. *Canadian Journal of Applied Physiology*, 26: 161–216.

Warburton, D.E.R., Nicol, C.W., & Bredin, S.S.D. (2006) Health benefits of physical activity: the evidence. *Canadian Medical Association Journal*, 174: 801–809

Weltman, A., Matter, S., & Stamford, B.A. (1980) Calorie restriction and/or mild exercise: Effect on serum lipids and body composition. *American Journal of Clinical Nutrition* 33: 1002–1009.

Winget, C.M., DeRoshia, C.W., and Holley, D.C. (1985) Circadian rhythms and athletic performance. *Medicine and Science in Sport and Exercise*, 17, 498–516.

Wolff, I., van Croonenborg, J.J., Kemper, H.C., et al. (1999) The effect of exercise training programs on bone mass: a meta-analysis of published controlled trials in pre- and postmenopausal women. *Osteoporosis International*, 9: 1–12.

Index

About the Authors

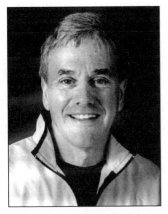

Robert Portman, Ph.D., has pioneered our understanding of how nutrition can enhance sports performance and improve weight management. As CEO and founder of Pacific Health Laboratories, Dr. Portman, who holds 11 patents, directed cutting-edge research that led to the development of novel nutritional formulas, which were shown to extend athletic endurance, speed muscle recovery, stimulate muscle growth, and activate the body's natural appetite control mechanisms. Dr. Portman is a sought-after lecturer who has authored hundreds of articles on nutrition. He has served as a nutritional consultant to many individual Olympic and professional athletes and sports teams. He is currently managing director of Signal Nutrition, a nutrition technology research and development company.

Along with Dr. Ivy, Dr. Portman coauthored *Nutrient Timing* (2004) and *The Performance Zone* (2004). The impact of *Nutrient Timing* on the entire spectrum of sports nutrition has been dramatic. The core principles outlined in the book are now part of the regular regimen of athletes and teams ranging from high school to professional.

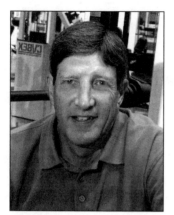 **John Ivy, Ph.D.**, is one of the preeminent exercise physiologists in the world. As head of the Department of Kinesiology at the University of Texas, and holder of the Teresa Lozano Long Endowed Chair, Dr. Ivy's research has advanced our understanding of how muscles work and how nutritional supplementation can improve muscle performance. As the author of over 150 scientific papers and numerous book chapters, Dr. Ivy's research has provided the underpinning for many practical and conceptual advances in our understanding of exercise physiology.

Dr. Ivy is frequently interviewed in print and on TV on issues involving exercise and fitness and has consulted for many commercial companies on sports nutrition. He is a Fellow of the International Society of Sports Nutrition, the American Academy of Kinesiology, and the American College of Sports Medicine, and is a recipient of the college's prestigious Citation Award.

In 2004, Dr. Ivy collaborated with Dr. Portman on *Nutrient Timing*, which has been called "the next important nutritional concept in the 21st century." In this book, the authors laid out a revolutionary system that adds the missing dimension to optimum sports nutrition—the dimension of time.

NUTRIENT TIMING
THE FUTURE OF SPORTS NUTRITION
John Ivy Ph.D. & Robert Portman, Ph.D.

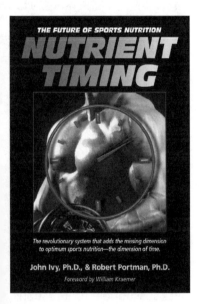

THE FUTURE OF SPORTS NUTRITION

NUTRIENT TIMING

The revolutionary system that adds the missing dimension to optimum sports nutrition—the dimension of time.

John Ivy, Ph.D., & Robert Portman, Ph.D.
Foreword by William Kraemer

Anyone who is serious about weight training has probably experienced the "plateau phenomenon"—that is, when despite training harder and consuming extra protein, you just don't get the strength and power gains that you want. For the last ten years, sports nutrition has focused on what to eat. The latest research from leading sports-science labs now shows that when you eat may be even more important.

Nutrient Timing adds the dimension that has been missing from sports nutrition: time. By timing the intake of specific nutrients to the muscle's twenty-four-hour growth cycle, an athlete can activate his or her body's natural anabolic agents to increase muscle growth and gain greater muscle mass than was ever thought possible.

Nutrient Timing will show readers how they can actually sculpt a better body with more lean muscle mass, less fat, and more power without changing their exercise program or even their total caloric intake.

$14.95 U.S. • TRADE PAPERBACK • ISBN: 158-1-59120-141-0 • 224 PAGES

THE PERFORMANCE ZONE
Your Nutrition Action Plan for
Greater Endurance & Sports Performance
John Ivy Ph.D. & Robert Portman, Ph.D.

Every athlete, coach, and parent of a young athlete knows that nutrition can enhance sports performance. But few know exactly how to make this happen. *The Performance Zone* solves this problem. This book synthesizes the most sound and up-to-date science to provide a nutrition action plan that enables athletes to raise their athletic performance.

The authors provide simple, proven guidelines for fueling muscles during and after sports activity. Using these guidelines, athletes can increase their endurance and strength, reduce injuries and muscle soreness, bounce back faster after training and competition, and even be less susceptible to infections.

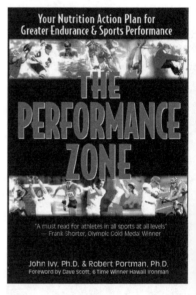

Since each sport has slightly different nutritional needs, *The Performance Zone* includes sports-specific nutrition tips from elite athletes, leading coaches, nutritionists, and exercise physiologists in the major individual and team sports.

$10.95 U.S. • TRADE PAPERBACK • ISBN: 158-1-59120-148-9 • 144 PAGES

For more information or to see our entire line of superior health titles, please visit www.basichealthpub.com